Induced Abortion and Spontaneous Early Pregnancy Loss - Focus on Management

Edited by Igor V. Lakhno

Published in London, United Kingdom

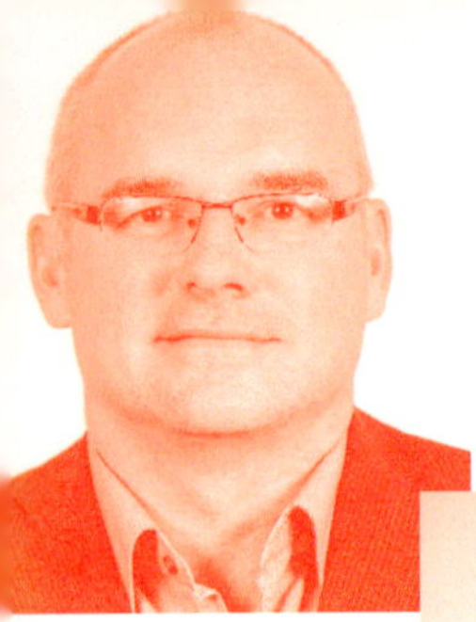
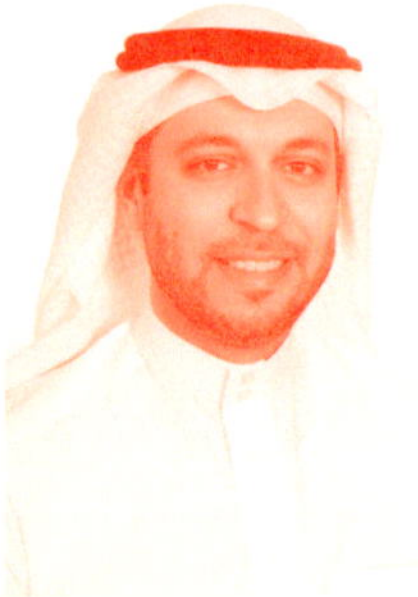
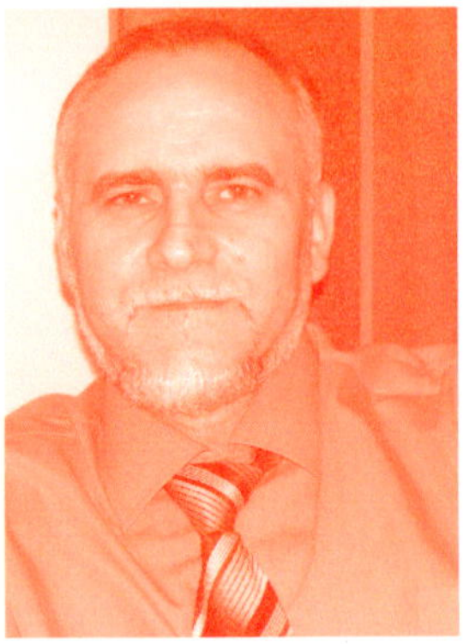
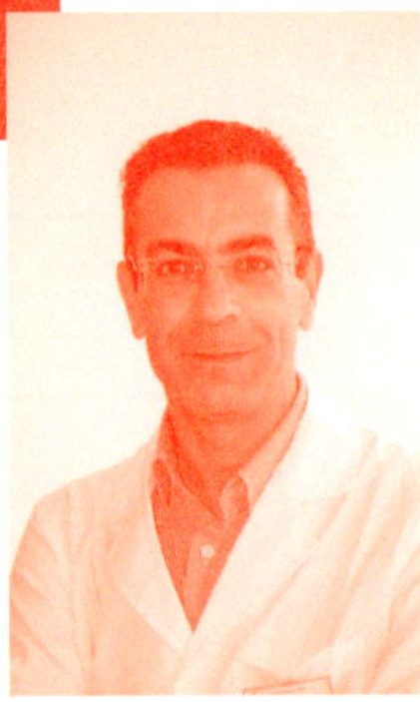
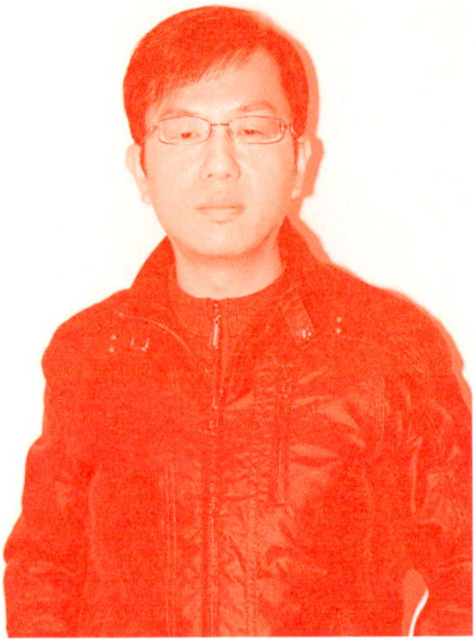
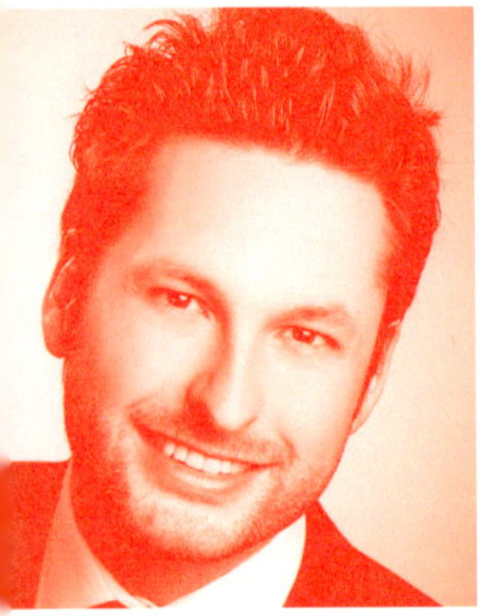
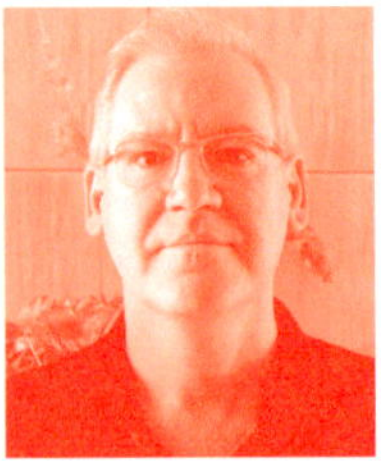

IntechOpen

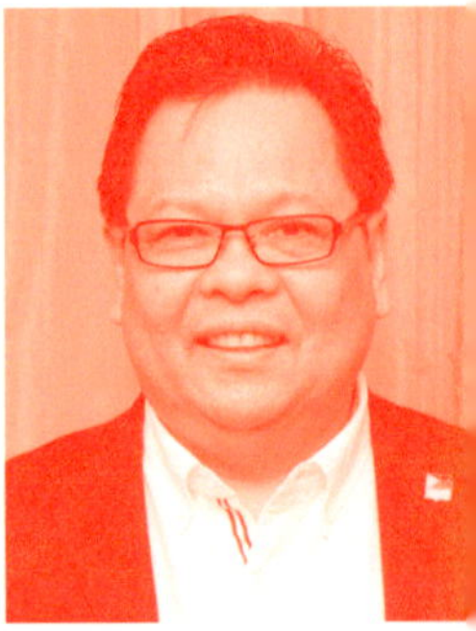
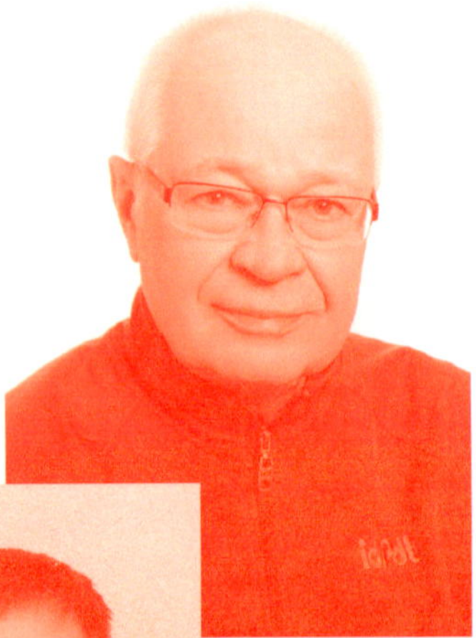
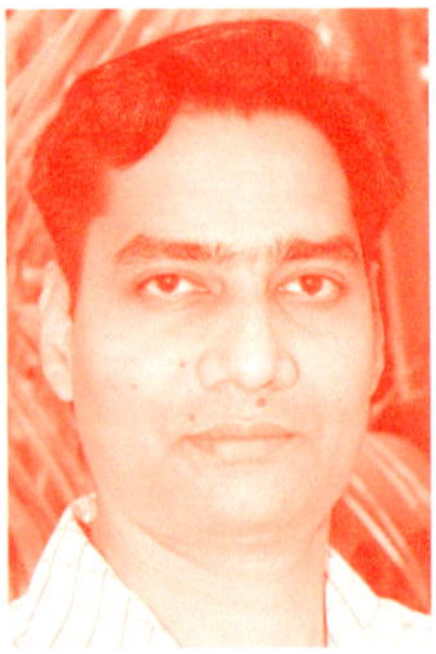
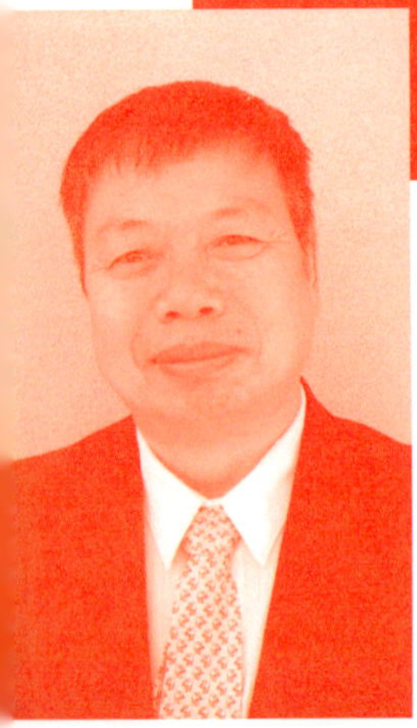
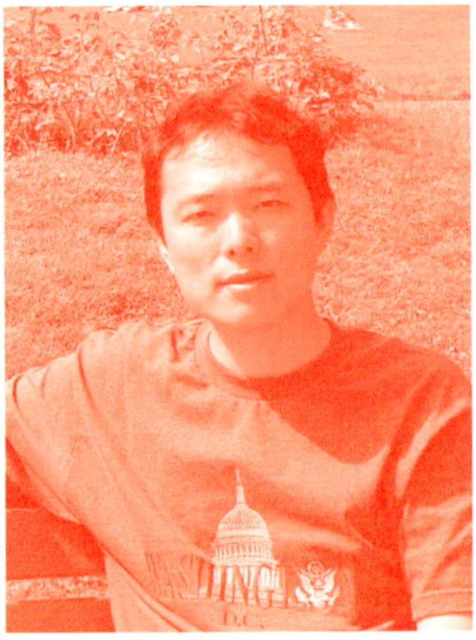
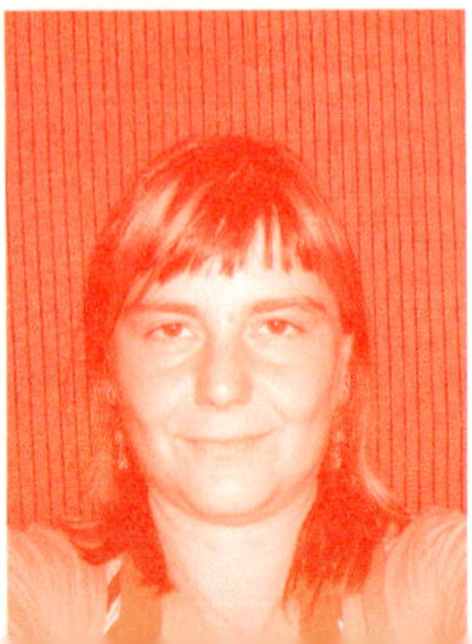

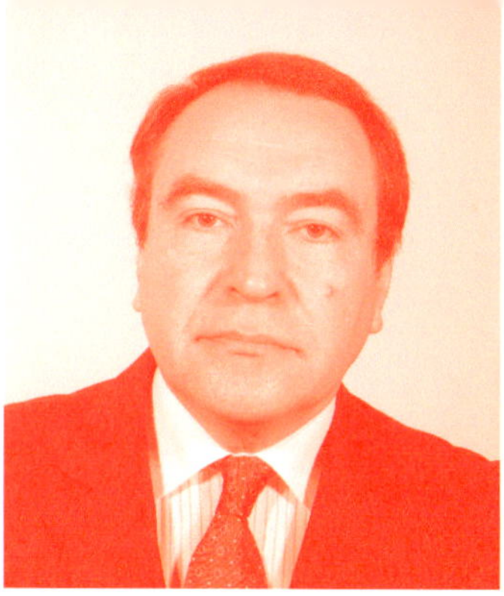
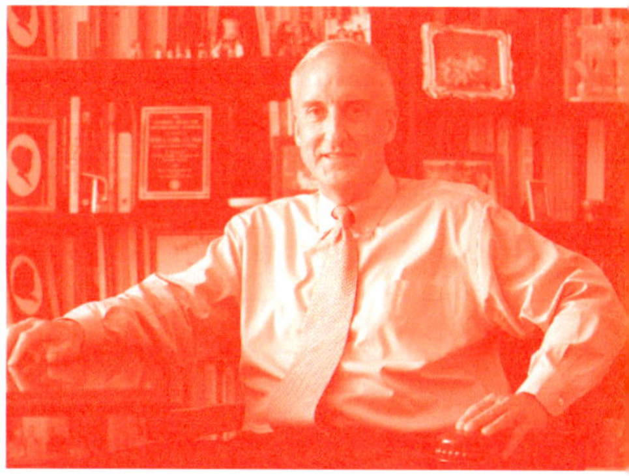
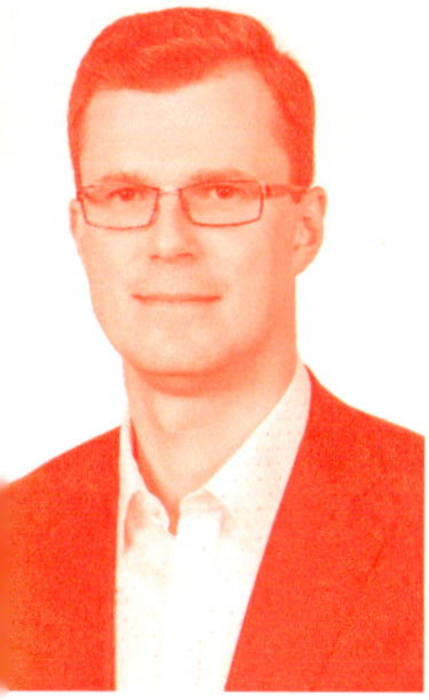
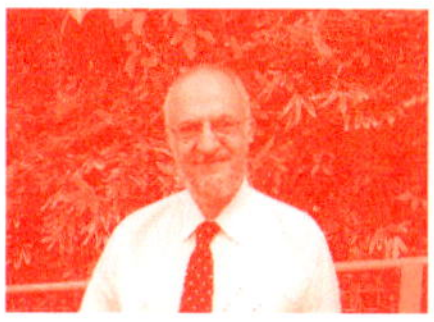
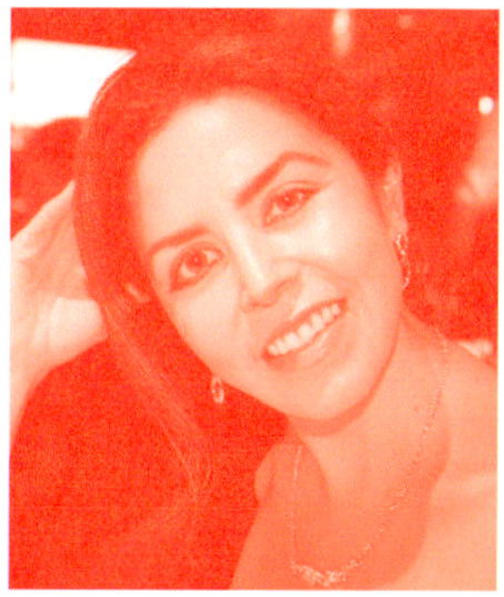

Supporting open minds since 2005

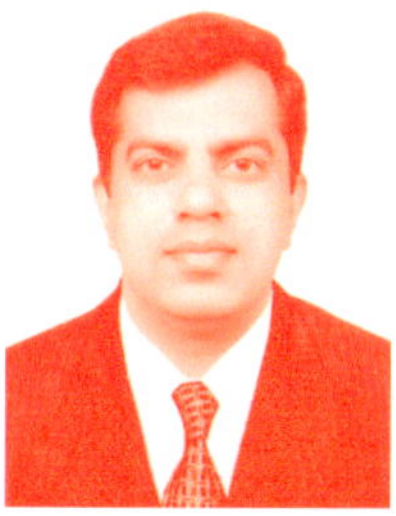
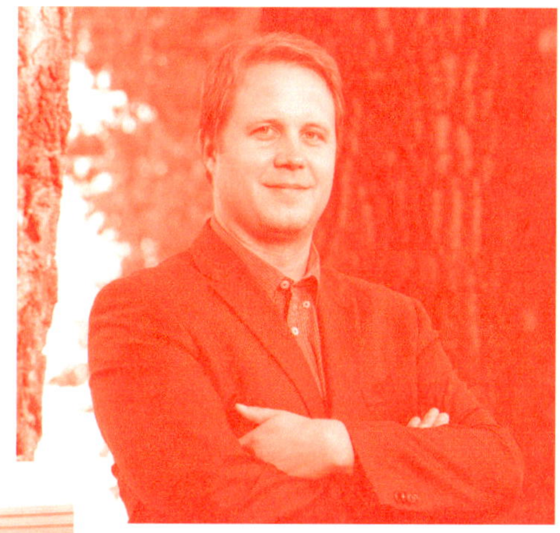
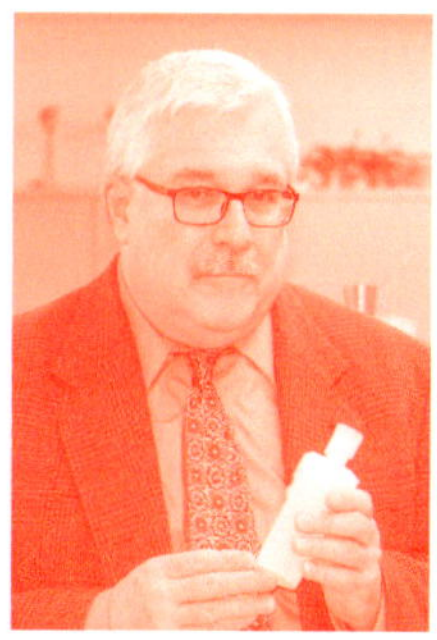
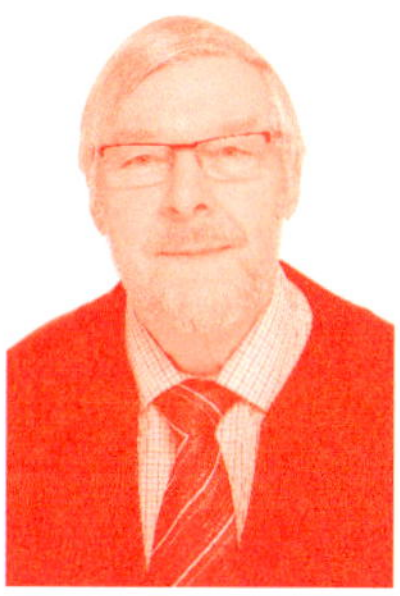
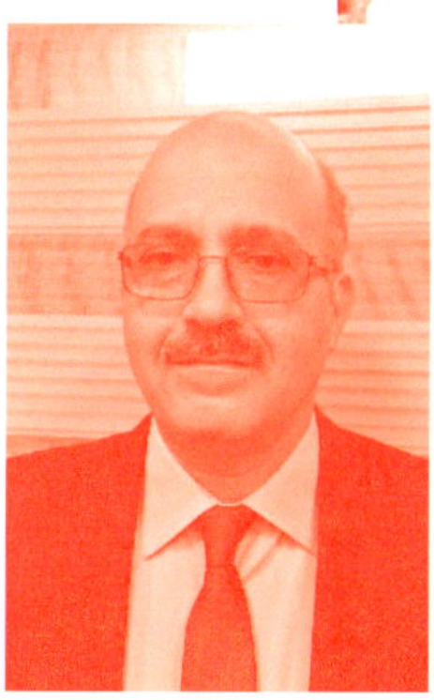
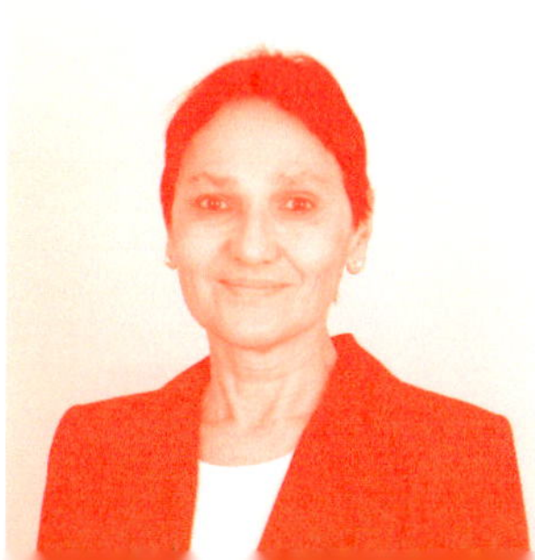
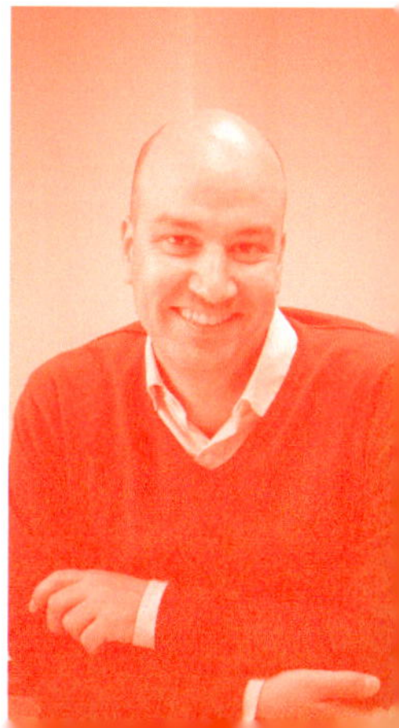

Induced Abortion and Spontaneous Early Pregnancy Loss - Focus on Management
http://dx.doi.org/10.5772/intechopen.77791
Edited by Igor V. Lakhno

Contributors
Wei-Hong Zhang, Jinlin Liu, Yvon Englert, Panagiotis Tsikouras, Theodora Deftereou, Xanthoula Anthoulaki, Anastasia Bothou, Anna Chalkidou, Fotini Gaitatzi, Ioannis Tsirkas, Arsou Chalil Bourazan, Eirini Bampageorgaka, George Stanulov, Eleftherios Chatzimichael, Panagiotis Petsidis, Georgios Iatrakis, Stefanos Zervoudis, Maria Lambropoulou, Werner Rath, Georgios Galazios, Spyridon Michalopoulos, Galina Dikke, Vladimir Ostromensky, Affonso Renato Meira, Jiřina Kocourková, Aleksandar Ljubic, Dzihan Abazovic, Andrea Pirkovic, Andjela Perovic, Dusica Ljubic

First published in London, United Kingdom, 2020 by IntechOpen
IntechOpen is the global imprint of INTECHOPEN LIMITED, registered in England and Wales, registration number: 11086078, 7th floor, 10 Lower Thames Street, London, EC3R 6AF, United Kingdom
Printed in Croatia

British Library Cataloguing-in-Publication Data
A catalogue record for this book is available from the British Library

Additional hard and PDF copies can be obtained from orders@intechopen.com

Induced Abortion and Spontaneous Early Pregnancy Loss - Focus on Management
Edited by Igor V. Lakhno
p. cm.
Print ISBN 978-1-78985-387-2
Online ISBN 978-1-78985-388-9
eBook (PDF) ISBN 978-1-78984-439-9

For EU product safety concerns:
IN TECH d.o.o., Prolaz Marije Krucifikse Kozulić 3, 51000 Rijeka, Croatia, info@intechopen.com or visit our website at intechopen.com.

Meet the editor

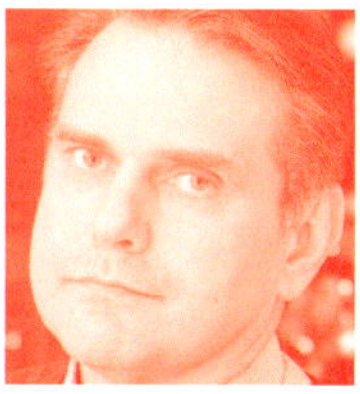

Igor V. Lakhno, MD (1994), PhD (1999), DSc (2019), is a professor at the Department of Obstetrics and Gynecology, Kharkiv National VN Karazin University, Ukraine. When a post-diploma student he graduated from an international training course on reproductive medicine and family planning held in Debrecen University (Hungary). His research interests include reproductive health, obstetrics, medical complications of pregnancy, fetal and maternal health, and gynecology. He is the author of about 200 printed works with many published in high-impacted journals and Scopus and Web of Science databases. He has participated as a speaker in several international conferences and congresses. Igor Lakhno is an editorial and reviewer board member of several scientific journals: *Health of Woman*, *Emergency Medicine*, and others.

Contents

Preface

Fertility regulation is a problem that is essential for life itself. The history of contraception has a strong relation to growing public interest. Induced abortion was formerly the only option and the main method of family planning. The negative attitude of society and religion to artificial abortion has a dramatic impact on its rate of reduction. The invention of hormonal contraception was one of the main events of the last century. It is contrary to human biology but hormonal contraception is the method of choice in Europe. The improved demographical situation in China over the last few decades has surprisingly increased the total level of induced abortions, but the involvement of the population in family planning is twice as high. The short- and long-term consequences of abortion on maternal and offspring health are still an issue. The decrease in the artificial abortion rate was found to be associated with improved maternal and perinatal outcomes. Therefore, the continuing battle against artificial abortion is an effective measure for the protection of female reproductive health.

The book contains fundamental data on the physiology of early gestation. The authors summarize theories to explain the pathogenesis of spontaneous abortion. Fetal and newborn health is known to be critically dependent on the intrauterine period of life. The fetal programming concept is based on the speculation that abnormal uteroplacental hemodynamics spreads a negative effect on fetal development and further diseases during postnatal life. Therefore, this book emphasizes endometrial status during preconception and implantation. The relevant complication of disturbed trophoblastic invasion is miscarriage. Spontaneous abortions are possibly involved in human evolution. But habitual abortion is a reason for active management. This text, therefore, presents the total spectrum of preventive and therapeutical interventions. One of the novel methods is based on biotechnology—the use of frozen human blood cells. The management of uterine scar pregnancy enhances the clinically oriented expectations of a reader. The post-cesarean uterine scar is associated with an excessive trophoblastic invasion and severe uterine bleeding during a surgical abortion. Thus, practical recommendations for the management of uterine scar pregnancy that contribute to the reduction of life-threatening complications are also presented.

The complications of abortion are well known. But the modern system of management is critically dependent on the latest medical advances, which could provide a wanted, safe, and happy pregnancy. This impact captures the total spread and positive outcome of family planning services in the world. The final goal is female reproductive health protection. Our book is only a small step in the march towards further development of modern contraceptive technologies and medical methods of recurrent pregnancy loss prevention.

The growing interest from the medical community to the problem of artificial and spontaneous abortion has induced this book. It is aimed at the introduction of a modern system for the prevention of artificial abortion and early pregnancy loss.

This book includes a preface by the editor, followed by six chapters written by international experts, arranged in two parts. It will be of great interest to social workers, psychologists, general practitioners, and gynecologists.

Igor V. Lakhno MD, PhD, DSc
Professor of the Obstetrics and Gynecology Department,
Kharkiv National VN Karazin University,
Ukraine

Section 1

Historical Review and Modern Trends in the Prevention of Unwanted Pregnancy

Chapter 1

Provoked Abortion

Affonso Renato Meira

Abstract

The provoked abortion is seen in many different ways in various countries. The woman that is supposed to be the main character of unfolding this procedure is usually unable to request it. The doctor that should be focused on doing the diagnosis about what the patient really wants for herself is also unable to do it, even if it is the best way to treat the situation. The values of different cultures act as impediments through laws that are oriented by religious beliefs and moral definitions leading to difficulties in the abortion scenario. Some facts are quite clear relating the woman and the doctor, who are the characters on this medical action, and that many times these are stopped or punished when they decide for themselves about abortion. The chapter intends to discuss the problem in many of countries of different continents, which focus the position of the doctor.

Keywords: abortion, law, religion

1. Introduction

When approaching a phenomenon, it is advised to investigate first what is already known about the subject, with the concerns of not searching what was already found [1].

In search of past times and since abortion is known as it is, we can verify that time passed does not allow secure statements, once nothing has been done in inviolable registry. Going through history, the first difficulty presents regards in knowing alternatives that could have no value. The culture of the people that habit different areas was and is distinct, as occurs nowadays.

Regarding the abortion, in general considerations, we remain with little information about the people that came before the white ones. Those people presented their culture in different parts of the globe and still do in many different forms.

To make an analysis that allows reflecting, it is necessary to state some arguments [2]. In this way it is needed to remember throughout the centuries, since there is registry of men living in earth, the life has its origins considered as born from the holy whisper of gods. Gods, from different rituals, since the mystics, characteristic of non-writing cultures, to those who had improved communication, were found in temples. These several rituals comprehend the donation of offerings that went to the worship of life. Gods, even though, used to serve to the explanation, in a dogmatic wat, of what occurs in the supernatural, exactly about what's beyond the human knowledge. Despite that, more recently, going against what common faith states, it was said that men created god. This affirmation represents a materialistic and rational thinking, but that loses most of the belief that humanity had in the past centuries since men are on this world.

For more that the scientific knowledge brings discoveries about how men got to this current situation, it's beginnings, which kind of evolution is possible from what type of life, questions that come along with controversy. It is possible to say that always, since the beginning of the concern with life, men wanted to know the world and its origin on earth, although there never was a moment in which we could delimitate precisely the appearance of men. In search of this, bonding, which can characterize, according with the theory of evolution, the passage of ancestral to the current men, is made every day, but what bonds the past and present is still missing. Those who, though rationally, based on scientific values have the position regarding men and its presence, which emerged producing conflicts in the middle of the nineteenth century. Recent ideas, if compared to other periods of humanity, have a strong force of modernity and to those who have higher study degrees. It is a reason that contradicts faith. The scientists from distinct backgrounds discuss with the believers from different religions [3].

In the holy bible, the ancient testimony, in the first book of Pentateuch, the book of origins, Genesis, it is written "In the beginning god created the sky and the earth," and the following can be found in the same book: "Let us make man in our image, after our likeness. And let them have dominion over the fish of the sea and over the birds of the heavens and over the livestock and over all the earth and over every creeping thing that creeps on the earth. So God created man in his own image, in the image of God he created him; male and female he created them."

According to the theory of evolution, proposed by Darwin, today considered by many, as completely verified in all of its aspects and meanings, the human beings are similar to one another and have a common ancestral at some point in the evolution. The origin of life occurred more than a billion years ago. Despite the studies and the information we have today, there is no existing evidence without questioning that allows us to understand undoubtedly those theories.

The theory of evolution has its acceptation in the elite society, for many academics and for scientist as to the lower layers of society who continue to believe in different gods stimulated by sacerdotes that independently of faith had always one or more gods to worship. This discussion is fundamental, because it builds the opinions regarding the main subject or we cannot analyze the sacred aspects of life. It is polemic if the most important is the holiness of life or its qualities. This brings together with what Engelhardt said "A moral life is lived in two different dimensions." Aside from any religious position, mainly through the catholic church, some incongruence is revealed between those that are against the possibility of freedom for abortion but accept other technics of assisted reproduction in which the embryo is discarded [4].

Besides different points of view, it is needed to bear in mind the role of women in society; it varies a lot as to where those societies are located. In those societies the culture reserves women a position, a role, and ways to behave in different ways. Meanwhile in occidental society, the role of women and their position include the possibility for them to achieve or to compete with the highest rank in politics as occurs in Argentina, Germany, Chile, France, Brazil, England, and/or the United States of America, to number a few; in other oriental countries, women are not given the rights to stay on the same level as their husband and friends, and they are also prohibited of going to the beach with swim clothes. The Islamic countries request women to cover their faces with a piece of cloth. The abortion position in the societies varies as time goes by, as the behavior of women varies as to what is imposed by the culture [5].

In all events that concern health issues, abortion gets highlighted for the difficulty in minimizing its impact on society. The problem of abortion presents difficulty in dialogue, once it presents very different opinions. In different societies ideals in relation to abortion are found; therefore, it's happening in the necessary conditions is having in mind health and always attending the religious prejudice, ethical and legal, although the standard behavior shows that the confrontation with the required level by society is inevitable, usually confronting law, health, religion, and ethics.

Looking in history for reference in the subject of abortion, we can find Hebrew had a code that got to the point of punishing those who practiced the abortion until the point of death. In Greek mythology we can find a quote by Aristotle that, in the beginning, was against the abortion and then agreed with the procedure if the embryo was found dead. Hippocrates—father of medicine—in reality was the precursor of medical ethics and was the author of the oath that doctors must follow, in which the practice of abortion is prohibited. In the oath of Hippocrates created before Christ, it is found "I shall not give women none abortive substance." In the Code of Hammurabi, the abortion is also punished. In Sparta, the abortion was forbidden in reason of the necessity of men to take charge of internal security and to build an army to intervene in times of war.

The question of abortion became a big theme when Saint Augustine pronounced about it and after Saint Tomas of Aquino differentiated the formed fetus and the fetus under formation. In the Roman Empire, the question was also reached.

Throughout the eighteenth century despite the little interest that abortion had in society, the practice was denied, mainly in reason of the scientific knowledge that were deployed, in the seventeenth and the eighteenth century, new bases leading to the fetus being recognized as an entity autonomously bring religious statements to echo in legislation.

With the French revolution and the beginning of the new nation, the wars, the plague, and the geographical discoveries, new changes occurred in the occidental world; the population growth started to go slower, meanwhile the necessity to keep a big army grew. The life of men was very important and the act of pregnancy was patriotic [5].

The position of abortion, in these societies, varied in distinct times, as the behavior of women varies for what is imposed by societies' culture.

The contradiction concerning the abortion obeys to these difficulties. The practice of abortion woke up all sorts of attention according to the cultural background. It is a subject that brings to the same place not only the professionals of health but also a quantity of academics of other disciplines such as lawyers, moralists, economists, legislators, judges, religious, and many others that at some point and for some reason found their selves discussing the subject.

The provoked abortion can be made under the coverage of medical sciences and with the approval of society or in an occasion that it is going against the law or other social values, an attitude that the community considers illegal. In this case the subject to be approached is whether the abortion provoked is under the coverage of the local community or if it is illegal, and in that way the prohibition makes shady to understand the circumstances under which the abortion is made.

Despite being a problem of medical practice, the procedure itself does not worry doctors, when taking good care of the environment and the patient, the result is mostly very positive [6].

The technics and the preparation of the environment are known in various types of medical school existing around the globe. The most concerning is the decision with the interruption of the pregnancy.

We need to have in mind that the one who desires the pregnancy does not wish to abort it and the one who desires the abortion does not wish the child; medicine is not against the abortion; nor the women nor the doctor is obligated to follow the procedure; who decides to follow the steps of this event is society.

The medical school presents two views of how to concretize the procedure: the one that involves taking medicine and a chirurgical one.

The procedure involving medicine is made through the oral use of a pill that will cause the fetus to be expelled which must be consumed as soon as possible to the event of pregnancy. In this way independent of medical recommendation, the pill may be bought from a drugstore. In many countries it is known as the "next-day pill." The drug is impregnated with levonorgestrel 1500 mcg taken in only one dose.

The chirurgical procedure is always provoked or induced, for medical or legal reasons. For that matter, the chirurgical abortion must be made as soon as possible, before the twelfth week of pregnancy in a sterilized environment as a chirurgical room, equipped with all the necessary tools. The patient needs to be examined carefully and must be submitted to pre-anesthesia and then be hospitalized and then submitted to anesthesia. According to the state of the women, the anesthesia can be done via oral or intravenous. It is, therefore, a hospital procedure. The withdrawal of the fetus is done through intrauterine vacuum aspiration, with a maximum from 12 to 14 weeks of pregnancy of the patient. Dilatation and curettage method, if still practiced, should be changed to aspiration. Between those methods the cut is used in the beginning of the pregnancy. A scraper is inserted into the woman's womb to separate the fetus into pieces that produces a lot of bleeding. Another way of producing the abortion is via applying a salty substance directly to the fetus that in the following hours will lose all its vital functions.

The chirurgical abortion must always be made by a doctor capable of the procedure, in a controlled chirurgical environment, and the conditions of health of the patient must be known. Aside from all innumerous aspects of culture and medical values, the doctor can under its own religious, ethics, and legal aspects take part in the event.

The legislation also has to take care of other important aspects as quality of social life. The legislation in many countries restricts abortion, and it sometimes allows it in two special punctual occasions: when it came from a raping situation or when there is no other way of saving the pregnant woman. The judicial system already discussed and decided in some societies to allow the procedure of abortion in those occasions when the fetus is anencephalic and when the fetus is microcephalic.

Social question to the women for many reasons may result that they cannot provide conditions for their children, they cannot keep the pregnancy, and they will have to interrupt it, but in many places it is forbidden.

Women without a partner, women abandoned by their partner, women whom the partner does not recognize the pregnancy, women without a partner that will not have the conditions to raise a child, women that have doubts of the pregnancy's paternity, women expelled from their house by their own family, children that will not know their father for many reasons, women that have no condition of recognizing the father, incestuous relationships, cases in which the anticonception measures failed, and many other possible scenarios push women into abortion. Women and children born in those conditions are often led to social discrimination that those who chose the legal or illegal abortion will not suffer [7]. In this way, as most of legislation, the norms and the laws are produced and made by men that take care of these aspects of human life since conception, laws that rule many but made by few.

The religious values varies with each faith and profundity of the same doctor and patient. The ethical values depend on what was established by the medical associations existing in the community, but legal values must be carefully obeyed in reason of being expressed in laws that define the doctor's behavior and the patient at the time of the intervention to provoke the abortion. These restrictions are extremely variable and have vast extension through different countries.

In most of the countries of the world, specially in the occidental world, the product of the composition in the parliaments shows a mix on restricted proposals in the subject of abortion.

There are also nations that have liberated entirely the abortions according to the pregnancy time. In general, from 12 until 24 weeks of pregnancy, the abortion is legal. In other counties, the abortion if emerged from a raping situation will not be criminalized. The incestuous is also considered, in many places as a sufficient act for the abortion to be made.

Mostly the doctors' point of view stands, therefore, when a woman is in risk or when there is no other way of saving the life of the pregnant, as a possibility that permits the conclusion of the abortion. Still as a medical factor, an anomaly of the fetus, case of anencephalic fetus or microcephalus cases, permits the procedure.

Those legislations normally come from the parliament that decides, in many times, a part of what is practiced inside the country. It is good to always remember that the higher institutions as supreme courts or superiors are legitimated in their competence to establish reasons not to punish a criminal who have practiced the abortion.

The abortion being spontaneous, or induced, via medicine or chirurgical is an act that occurs in women and that requires in modern society the presence of doctors.

The decision in society to liberate or repress depends on various aspects, inclusively the scientific [7].

The position of the government in considering laicism or religious is a main factor, whereas the religious states depend on the religious perspective on the abortion, and if it condemns the abortion, there is not much to be done. About this argument that at some point seems dubious, there is the example of catholic church in the state of Vatican. In the catholic doctrine, abortion is a sin that those who conclude it will suffer and be expelled automatically. The forgiveness to this sin is only in the hands of the pope to whom he delegates this act.

Societies dominated by tyrannies also take position to present restrictions for women to come forward looking for medical attention even when the abortion is spontaneous. El Salvador country in Central America condemns the death of women that goes through abortion to which there is no condition to prove if it was provoked or spontaneous.

These are extreme examples of what happens in most of countries that, if the abortion is not entirely liberated, do not repress entirely it [3].

Even if the scientific knowledge does interfere in the parliament proposals, the political struggle will be the one to try to balance the value of public opinion. The ways people are represented vary a lot. The values of medicine such as the wishes of women are listened and mixed with religious doctrines, social-economic conditions, population characteristics, political party orientation, and many other factors that influence the congressman opinions.

The chirurgical abortion is not possible obeying only the doctors' view; before that it is needed to have the possibility of attending the religious values, the ethical, and essentially the laws.

As every legislation, norms and laws are produced and elaborated by men that take care of aspects of human life since its conception satisfice many but not all.

Rodrigo Torres, a judge, in an article stated comparing legislations from several nations in the twenty-first century and showed a panorama of the situation in the European Union [4]:

A. Prohibition without any exceptions: Malta

B. Abortion permitted if asked by the women, with any time determinate in the pregnancy (90 days to 4 weeks): United Kingdom, Netherlands, Sweden, Romania, Denmark, Lithuania, Check Republic, Slovakia, Greece, Hungry, Belgium, Bulgaria, France, Germany, Latvia, Estonia, Portugal, Slovenia, Austria, and Italy

C. Abortion permitted in accordance to the risk of life of the pregnant: United Kingdom, Denmark, Sweden, Latvia, Poland, Slovenia, Austria, Check Republic, Slovakia, Romania, Cyprus, Greece, Hungary, Spain, Portugal, France, Germany, Lithuania, Estonia, Luxemburg, and Ireland (including risk of suicide)

D. Abortion permitted in reason of risk of life of the pregnant, with some time determinate in pregnancy: Netherlands and Finland

E. Abortion permitted in case of risking the life of the pregnant within any time: Denmark, Slovenia, Austria, Check Republic, Slovakia, Romania, Cyprus, Hungary, Italy, France, and Germany

F. Abortion permitted when the pregnancy results of rape or sexual crime, always: Romania, Cyprus, Greece, Germany, and Hungary

G. Abortion permitted when the pregnancy results of a rape or another sexual crime within some time of pregnancy (from 90 days to 28 weeks): Denmark, Finland, France, Spain, Belgium, Poland, Italy, Luxemburg, Portugal, Latvia, Lithuania, Netherlands, and Estonia

H. Abortion permitted when there is a problem with the fetus formation, within any time: Netherlands, Denmark, Sweden, Finland, Latvia, Estonia, and Luxemburg

I. Abortion permitted for social economic reasons within any time: Netherlands, Finland, Italy, France, and Luxemburg

In this work it is also possible to find considerations about Latin America.

Cuba in 1965 legalized abortion until 12 weeks of pregnancy and maintained an abortion percentage under 21 in every thousand of women in reproductive age, 10 points under the regional average.

Chile, El Salvador, Nicaragua, and the Dominican Republic criminalized abortion without exceptions. Honduras, following the code of medical ethics, allows the abortion to save the life of the pregnant.

Argentina, Costa Rica, Venezuela, Peru, and Paraguay admit the abortion to save the life of the pregnant; being that in Argentina, the permission also covers women that are not capable of perceiving the reality, and in Venezuela it is allowed to protect the honor of men and women.

Uruguay, Colombia, Equator, Bolivia, Mexico, Panama, and Guatemala admit the abortion in cases of rape and incestuous pregnancy; Uruguay also allows the procedure of economical struggle and Colombia, Mexico, and Panama when there is a formation problem within the fetus. Brazil maintains the criminalization of abortion without punishment when resulted from rape or when there is no other way of saving the woman's life; in this way the anencephalic abortion is not punished agreeing to the supreme court's decision. The United States of America in the constitution liberates the abortion procedure, but there is some bureaucracy in different states.

Other countries not remembered could be brought to this subject. It is the case of those who hardened the laws against abortion. Between these is Japan. Turkey is where the abortion is permitted with pregnancy until the tenth week, and the decision is of the women. In Israel, the abortion is permitted when it presents physical or psychological risk to the women, in cases of problems in fetus formation and humanitarian reasons. The pregnancy of a second son or a non-authorized pregnancy, in China, makes women to be obligated to abort.

In Russia, abortion is legal until the twelfth week of pregnancy. In 1920, Russia became the first country to legalize abortion in all circumstances, whereas through the twentieth century, the legislation concerning abortion in the country was modified, and its prohibition came back in 1936, remaining this way until 1954. According to data from the United Nations, Russia has the highest number of abortions per women in fertile age of the world, between 15 and 40 years, with about 1.3 million abortions (absolute number) realized per year, which is about 53.7 abortions per 1000 women. The Italian legislation before 1978 used to consider a crime interruption in pregnancy, but with the implementation of law 194, on that year, the voluntary abortion was decriminalized, permitting it until the third month of the pregnancy in public hospitals in Italy and in the fourth or the fifth month in case of therapeutic nature (when there is risk for the mother and in detection of bad formation and other anomalies). In this country a higher percentage of doctors, obstetrics, and anesthetists can be found, about 70%, that deny making the procedure.

The abortion in New Zealand was legalized, since 1977, until 20 weeks of pregnancy and after 20 weeks, if impacting the women's health. The legislation requires that after 20 weeks the abortion needs to be made in public hospitals. In Australia the abortion is legalized since 1970. The increasing number of women going through the procedure made the government to launch a public policy to decrease the number.

In Mozambique it was regulated by a law and was permitted only in case of risking the pregnant women, in case of rape, until the tenth week. The law was approved by the president in 2014.

During the Mandela government, in the Republic of South Africa, the abortion was legalized. There are private clinics, but the government offers the service for free. Until the twelfth week, the procedure is through pill taking. In the African continent besides the Republic of South Africa and Mozambique, Green Cape and Tunisia are other countries that have a legislation about abortion.

The quote of the happenings in relation to different countries with very different religious backgrounds, varying the geographic location and political organization, allows us to understand that the liberation or restriction of abortion depends more on the social and political field than in the scientific field. The chirurgical risk of the procedure is very little.

The attention to the legislation in each country is the first step to take when approaching the subject and the procedure having in mind the possible punishments. On different countries, the legislation comes slowly changing, not only following the advance on medical sciences but modifying the laws of social behavior varying in each society [8].

The religious aspects have to always be considered between the patient and the doctor, their beliefs, and how society refers to it. Contradictions are found within followers of different religions that spread across the globe. A rough calculation expects more than 3000 sects with doctrines and dogmas, its particularities, and the essence not differing much [5].

In reality the religion that affects most the occidental world and strongly present in Latin countries is Catholicism, side to side to other many doctrines that are influenced by Catholicism.

In the occidental world, the Judaic religion is also disseminated that finds its center in Jerusalem and the state of Israel.

The oriental countries are followers of other religions such as Buddhism, Hinduism, and Islamism. The Buddhism and its sects have a high location in Japan. Islamism is prominent in Iran and in other Arabic countries. Hinduism is situated mainly in India, Nepal, Pakistan, and Sri Lanka. Other sects and religious doctrines are found and spread throughout the world with pastors worshiping different theological thoughts with followers that also go in various ways.

Catholicism, as a religion, was dominated by the first 15,000 years in the occidental world after Christ. In 1517 Martin Luther, a Frey from the Saint Augustine, promoted a big movement breaking with the unity of the church. The reform brought to question social and political aspects of the society in Europe. In a bigger meaning, the reform refers to other movements within the catholic church, as Calvinism in Switzerland that originated the evangelic church and Henry VIII in England that derivate the Anglican Church. These movements brought the council of Trent, giving birth to an inside reform of the church. Nowadays with the presence of Pope Francis, there is a walk towards the proximity between those churches.

In the catholic religion, the practice of abortion is considered a capital sin leading those who practice to be expelled. The pope had the power to forgive after the abortion if the people regretted, truly delegated in November 2016 the grace of forgiving in all countries, as the bishops have done before him. In any way the abortion to the Catholics keeps being judged as a capital sin.

In opposition to the catholic church that its followers spread without any worrying of agglomerating, the followers of the Judaic religion conglomerate to build mutual help. In this way, the usual Jewish marriage is within the same religion. It is common for the Jewish colonies to have institutions such as hospitals to give services of health and schools for teaching, obeying religious aspects. In opposite of many other religions, the Jewish orthodox followers usually pay close attention to the religious traces. In Judaism it is considered that the fetus or the embryo has no condition of person before the birth. Inside the Jewish population of the world, it can be considered that an ethnic group has ethnical divisions, most being a result of geographical ramification of the Israeli population and independent evolving of the several Jewish communities around the world. Nowadays, manifestations of these ethnical differences in the Jewish community can be observed as cultural expressions of each place, such as linguistic differences. The ethnical division of Jews was into two main groups as to Ashkenazi and Sephardi. These two groups are characterized by locality of habiting. The Ashkenazi settled mostly in the Anglo-Germanic part of Europe. The Sephardi searched the Latin side, whereas the Misraim and the Teimanim are the "Yemenites that live in the oriental side of the world."

In what refers to abortion in the Jewish religion, if the embryo or the fetus presents a risk to the women, the abortion is allowed among the most orthodox groups, the conservative, and the reformers. Between the reformists the well-being (social and psychological conditions) can be considered to approval. As to the tradition of the Maimonides, in the twelfth century, if the embryo offers a risk to health, mental, or physical well-being of the woman, she can interrupt the pregnancy, as self-defense, as the embryo is considered an aggressor. The decision has to be made besides a rabbin. It is important to compare with Christianism the traditional Jewish religion does not allow that the individual decision of the women but her will has to be accompanied with the permission of a rabbin that in his wisdom will find what is moral and just.

On the Buddhist point of view, abortion is considered a homicide, although there could be various motivations to terminate pregnancy. If the motivation is a selfish unconcern, as to not wanting to take care of a baby, it becomes the hardest act in the eyes of Buddhism, because the motivation and the act are both destructive. In Buddhism, the motivation can also be positive. If the baby is very deformed or mentally insufficient, so wanting to prevent any further suffering, it is not condemned to abort considering the secondary vote of bodhisattva practiced by all Buddhists that the destructible act should not be avoided if the motivation is positive. The ethics here could also be questioned.

In another situation, in the case of risk to the mother during the pregnancy, many factors and circumstances come into play on the decision taking, being that it is defined by the karma that will be the judge of that action in another life depending on the consequences of the abortion. Beyond the causal motivation, the Buddhist teaches that the contemporary motivation (what an individual thinks about abortion) is also very important when justifying the abortion. In this way, it is important to a Buddhist, in the moment of the abortion, to have in mind the carrying thoughts. Some Buddhist traditions do make celebrations for the fetus. Supposedly, the realization of those ceremonies is extremely useful for the "soul" of the mother. A name is given to the fetus which is prayed for upon their lives. "The goal of the Buddhists is to achieve spiritual enhancement, the 'nirvana' estate of freedom from unhappiness and from the pain existing in the world, a spirituality of peace and happiness." Although there is no consensus on Buddhism as to abortion, most of its followers consider it a rupture in the flow of life. Traditional Buddhist sources, as to the monastic code, point that the destruction of deliberated life is a hard rupture of the traditional teachings. The actual Dalai Lama considers the abortion a mistake but considers that there are occasions that it is justified. Even though when the abortion is done to save the life of the woman, it is almost always seen as causing a suffering and negative karma.

The followers of Islamism, as to the Coran, condemn the action of killing; many stick to fanatic in following, for example, a war, as of not worrying to die, with the idea that will bring them in the presence of Allah. This fanatic position in good times reaches the belief of young boys that with some frequency explode bombs attached to their bodies, in crowded places with the intention of practicing terrorism and without fearing death. The main cause of condemnation of abortion among Muslims is in the historical roots.

Hinduism is a religion that has various gods that are venerated in different occasions and different places, in general, condemns the act of abortion.

Beyond these churches of the dominant point of view in the occidental world, as in the oriental world, other sects can be analyzed.

The church of Jesus Christ and the Saints in the Last Days, the Mormons, do not advice the procedure of abortion; they go against it. Although if the preservation of women health or the pregnancy is resulted from a rape case, in this manner to save the spiritual life of women, the procedure is permitted by the president of the church and then consulted by a doctor.

In the Anglican Church, many consider a point of view aside of the church's main decision. There is a permission for it to be done, despite many forbidding the abortion.

The Methodist church presumes that abortion is an extreme case, when there is a risk for the mother's life, because it should have the conditions to having more children and should also have the chance of taking care of the children already existing. It is admitted the possibility of abortion in pregnancy coming from a rape case if the woman does not wish to keep the pregnancy, considering that she was not given the choice of the sexual act, a point of view that goes against the holy spirit of the evangelic announced by Jesus Christ. The interruption of pregnancy in cases that medicine proves the unviability of the survival of the fetus is admitted, as it is the case of anencephalic fetus (fetus without encephalic mass that only remains alive as long as the maternal body is fed).

As to the Jehovah Testimonies, in what concerns the abortion, there is not a standard position generally considering that interrupting the pregnancy is a heavy sin and it is a killing of the fetus. The same position that the one adopted by society is legal and established as right is usually accepted.

The Universal Church of the Kingdom of God is an evangelical church, with its headquarters in the Salomon's Temple, in São Paulo, Brazil. Founded in the 9th of July of 1977 by Edir Macedo, it became one of the fastest growing religious groups in the world with approximately 6000 temples, 12,000 pastors, and 1.8 million followers around the country and 8 million around the world and 15,000 in 105 countries, being the most popular in Portuguese-speaking nations. It is one of the biggest religious organizations of Brazil and the twenty-ninth biggest church in followers of the world. In a public declaration made more than 10 years ago and recently reaffirmed, pastor Macedo clarifies: "I'm in favor of abortion. I'm in favor of women having the right to decide."

Sex and sexual pleasure are accepted as a desirable practice between Taoism and Confucianism. The practice must be observed with moderation and also the practice be considered in relation to reproduction and the abortion as an acceptable resource, although there are groups of Taoists aiming the preservation of life that have a vision against abortion.

Many of the native North American cultures have a woman-centered point of view when it comes to abortion, looking at it as a valid option. Other existing religions do not present followers in a considerable number that by occasion intervene or not in some way on abortion.

2. Final comment

After the passage of what occurs in most part of the world, in relation to what is necessary to know about the operation of the abortion, it is possible to consider that greater are the barriers to follow through with the procedure than they are to be stopped. Beyond that through the dialogue, the conclusion is reached that it is necessary to have optimal conditions to operate.

The first condition for an abortion to be provoked is the women's desire and that she fulfils the health conditions, time of pregnancy, age, and psychological conditions.

The second is the presence of a doctor capable of proceeding and authorized by the professional associations. Another condition is the existence of a local such as a hospital environment filled with the necessary tools and life support. As all those aspects related to the characters that agreed on the procedure are fulfilled, it is needed to have in mind the religious aspects too the involved and that those do not prohibit the event.

In the end, it is needed to verify the location, the city, and the country where it is intended to be practiced. The chirurgic procedure has appropriate laws for that manner and if they allow or prohibit it. If the abortion is punished without exceptions, it cannot be made. If it fills the exceptions, then it shall be done.

All of that shows that it is easier to understand and that it is harder to find an abortion that obeys all the laws, religious beliefs, and morality of the involved than it is to find a secure but illegal abortion.

Author details

Affonso Renato Meira
University of São Paulo, Brazil

*Address all correspondence to: ar.meira@terra.com.br

References

[1] Fernandes AG. Aborto; aspectos jurídicos e políticos. In: Martins IGS, Carvalho PB, editors. Inviolabilidade do Direito à Vida. São Paulo: Noeses; 2013. pp. 79-92

[2] Meira AR. Editorial da revista. Reprodução e Climatério. 2015;**30**(2). DOI: 10.1016/j.reclic 2015,09/003

[3] Meira AR. A incongruência no abortamento. Suplemento Cultural da Revista da APM. 2019. n°310

[4] Torres JHR. Abortos; artigos [Abortion]. São Paulo; 2016

[5] Meira AR. Abortion and Family Planning in Family Planning. London: IntechOpen; 2018. pp. 279-298

[6] Proença NG. Abortamento sim ou não? Suplemento da Revista da APM. 2019. n°309

[7] Meira AR. A Medicine e o abortamento. Suplemento Cultural da Revista da APM. 2018. n° 308

[8] Meira, A.R. Abortamento: Introducão e Perspectivas, New Academic Editions, Saarbrucken; 2017. p. 80

Chapter 2

Is Induced Abortion a Part of Family Planning in China?

Jinlin Liu, Yvon Englert and Wei-Hong Zhang

Abstract

Family planning policy is one of the basic policies in China. Since the founding of New China, it has gone through three stages during its development process, which include free fertility policy, one-child policy (including selective two-child policy), and universal two-child policy. The number of induced abortions in China has increased from 3,910,110 in 1971 to 9,626,731 in 2017, and the proportion of induced abortions in birth control surgeries of family planning in China has increased from 30.0% in 1971 to 50.6% in 2017. It is concluded that although induced abortion is not a part of the family planning policy of China, it has been a part of family planning services in China.

Keywords: family planning, induced abortion, policy, contraception, China

1. Introduction

As one of the basic policies in China, the family planning policy plays a vital role in regulating the fertility level of the population and the total population number. Before 2016, the one-child policy of China is well known all over the world due to its strict regulation and implementation. As one of the important means of birth control surgeries, many scholars think that induced abortion is a part of China's family planning policy and plays an important role during the implementation process of one-child policy. This chapter will make a macroanalysis of the history and current situation of the family planning policy and induced abortion in China and further analyze the relationship between them, thus to finally answer whether induced abortion is a part of family planning in China.

2. The history and current situation of the family planning policy in China

As is known to all, the family planning policy remains one of the basic policies in China. Actually, the family planning policy has existed since ancient China. Beginning with the establishment of Qin dynasty, the family planning policy was always implemented to encourage fertility from 221 BC to 617 AD. In Tang dynasty which was the height of feudal age, it had been a basic state policy to encourage fertility from 618 to 907 AD [1]. However, from then on, some scholars had begun to suggest to control the population growth speed.

Wang Fanzhi, who was a poet in the early period of Tang dynasty, was regarded as the first person to put forward that one couple should only have one child. In the

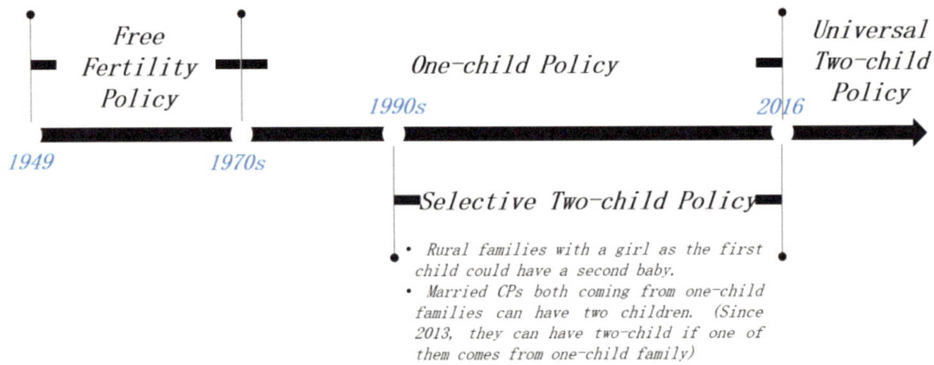

Figure 1.
Development process of family planning policy in China since 1949.

later dynasties of Song, Ming, and Qing, although there were no specific regulations in family planning policies, the governments did not encourage fertility. Ma Duanlin, a famous scholar in the end of the Song dynasty and the author of *Wenxian Tongkao*, put forward a relatively complete family planning theory which included fewer births, healthier births, and paying more attention to comprehensive population quality. And it was very similar with the modern population and family planning policy in China. Wang Meicun, the demographer in Qing dynasty and the author of *Yi Bing Ri Ji*, was regarded as the first person to put forward that the government should reduce its population birth rate. He put forward the strategy for controlling population growth by implementing drug abortion on women after the first child [2–4].

After the founding of the New China, with the changes of country situation, the China's family planning policy has gone through three big stages with a series of reforms [5]. **Figure 1** shows the development process of family planning policy in China since 1949.

1. The first stage was from the time of country founding to the early 1970s. Affected by the former Soviet Union's theory of encouraging population growth, the Great Leap Forward and the national famine from 1959 to 1961 in China and other factors, although the Chinese government advocated independent birth control, the society presented a trend of substantially fair fertility which has led to the rapid population growth [6].

2. The second stage was from the mid-1970s to late 1990s. The family planning policy was adopted by the Chinese Government in the mid- and late 1970s to respond to the challenge of China's enormous population. It was identified as one of the basic national policies in the 12th National Congress of the Communist Party of China and was written into the national constitution in December 1982. From then on, the family planning policy of advocating that one couple should only have one child was implemented forcibly to strictly control the population growth speed. In particular, the Chinese government relaxed the policy regulation in rural areas and allowed families with a girl as the first child to have a second child [7].

3. The third stage was from the early 2000s to date. With the continuous decline of population total fertility rate and serious challenge by the impending aging society, the Chinese government began to pay more attention on how to make adjustment on the family planning policy thus to promote population growth to a certain extent and change the imbalanced age structure of the population.

> In September 2002, the *Population and Family Planning Law of the People's Republic of China* came into effect. From then on, the Chinese government encouraged the couple who are both from one-child families to have two children. In November 2013, it was proposed to implement the policy of selective two-child policy in the *Decision of the Central Committee of the Communist Party of China on Some Major Issues Concerning Comprehensive Deepening the Reform*, which meant that the couple that as long as one of them was from the one-child family could have two children. However, it did not work well. Some scholars pointed out that China has fallen into the low fertility rate trap. In October 2015, the 18th Central Committee of the Chinese Communist Party decided to abolish the basic one-child policy and selective two-child policy and to replace them by a universal two-child policy which meant that every couple can have two children. The revised *Population and Family Planning Law of the People's Republic of China* has come into effect since January 1, 2016 [8–11].

In general, after being implemented for 40 years, the Chinese government considers the family planning policy to be a great success, because it has significantly reduced population growth. The fertility rate has dropped from 5.8 in the 1970s to 1.7 in 2013 [12]. China has entered the ranks of low-fertility-level counties. The ability and quality of family planning services are quickly upgraded. And it has significantly improved the population quality. However, the policy has its drawbacks. For instance, the age structure of population is unbalanced, the birth sex ratio is unbalanced, the population quality is different between urban and rural areas, etc. [13].

At present, besides the universal two-child policy, the Chinese family planning policy also includes some key aspects as follows:

First, in terms of the reproduction regulation, (1) family planning shall be implemented chiefly by means of contraception. The state creates conditions to ensure that individual citizens have the rights of informed choice to choose safe, effective, and appropriate contraceptive methods. When birth control operations are performed, the recipients' safety shall be ensured; (2) couples of reproductive ages shall conscientiously adopt contraceptive methods and accept technical services and guidance for family planning. Incidence of unwanted pregnancies shall be prevented and reduced; and (3) couples of reproductive ages who implement family planning shall receive the basic items of family planning technical services specified by the state for free.

Second, in terms of the family planning technical services, (1) the state establishes premarital healthcare and maternal healthcare systems, thus to prevent or reduce the incidence of birth defects and improve the health of newborns; (2) the governments at all levels shall take measures to ensure citizens' access to technical services for family planning in order to improve their reproductive health; and (3) persons who provide technical services for family planning shall give guidance in citizens who implement family planning in choosing the safe, effective, and appropriate contraceptive methods.

Third, the illegal behaviors include (1) illegally performing operations to family planning on other persons, (2) using ultrasonography or other techniques to identify fetal gender or to bring about sex-selective pregnancy termination for nonmedical purposes for other persons, and (3) providing a fake medical report or issuing a counterfeit certificate of family planning.

3. The history and current situation of induced abortion in China

Induced abortion is a concept of modern medicine which is different from spontaneous abortion. However, induced abortion has existed since ancient times in China. In ancient China, encouraging fertility is not only a kind of conception but also an official policy implemented by the rulers; thus the rulers were opposed to abortion. Since the Qin dynasty and Han dynasty, forced abortions of pregnant women or causing death by abortions would be regarded as criminal acts [14]. The earliest records about abortion in Chinese history began in the Han dynasty, and it had formed three kinds of abortion skills which included drug abortion, external force abortion, and acupuncture abortion. After the Tang dynasty and Song dynasty, due to the pressure of population growth, abortions had become a universal tendency in some areas, which finally led to the open and profession of abortion [15]. In the Qing dynasty, the Republic of China, and the early period of New China during twentieth century, abortion is still regarded as a criminal act which was clearly specified in related criminal laws. At the beginning of New China, the central government strictly restricted sterilization and induced abortion. However, in August 1953, with the promulgation of the Guide for Contraception and Induced Abortion in China, induced abortion had been legalized basically. Since 1979, the crime of abortion had been abolished from the new criminal law of China [16]. At present, abortion in Taiwan of China still remains a crime unless during emergency [17].

In general, as shown in **Figure 2**, according to the statistical results in *China Health Statistics Yearbook 2018*, the overall level of induced abortion of family planning in China presents a trend of ups and downs from 1971 to 2017. In 1971, the number of induced abortions was 3,910,110, and it reached the highest level in history in 1983 with 14,371,843. Then the number was maintained between 600 and 800 million in the twentieth century. At present, the number of induced abortions in China was 9,626,731 in 2017, which was about 2.5 times than that in 1978. **Figure 3** shows the proportions of induced abortions in birth control survey of family planning in China from 1971 to 2017. It presents an overall trend of gradual growth from 30.0% in 1971 to 50.6% in 2017.

In addition, there are some other research results about the induced abortion situation in China [18–22]. First, induced abortion among females presents a younger trend. The age of women who had induced abortions is mainly distributed from 20 to 29 years old, and those who are under 25 years account for nearly half. Second, the proportion of induced abortions of young unmarried women ranges from 20 to 30% among all induced abortions, and their age are basically under 24 years old. Third, among married women who have induced abortions, the peak

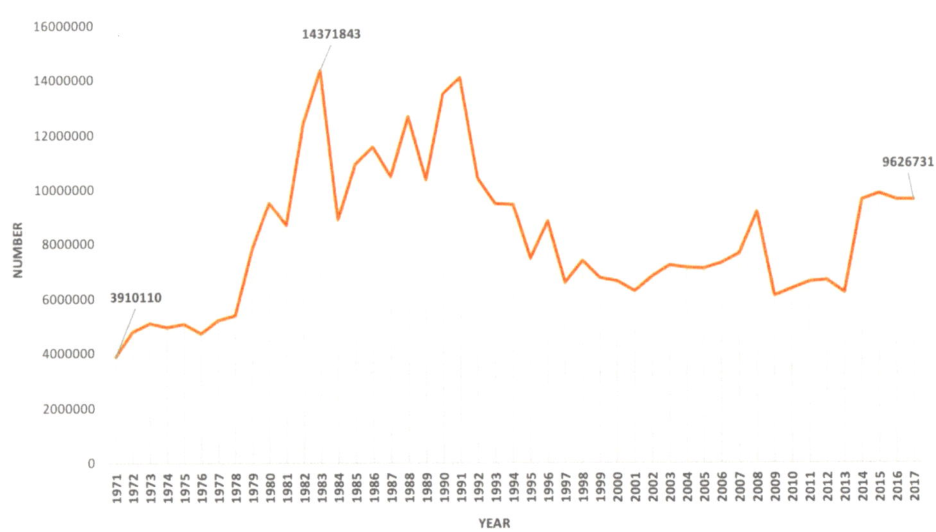

Figure 2.
Number of induced abortions within family planning services in China.

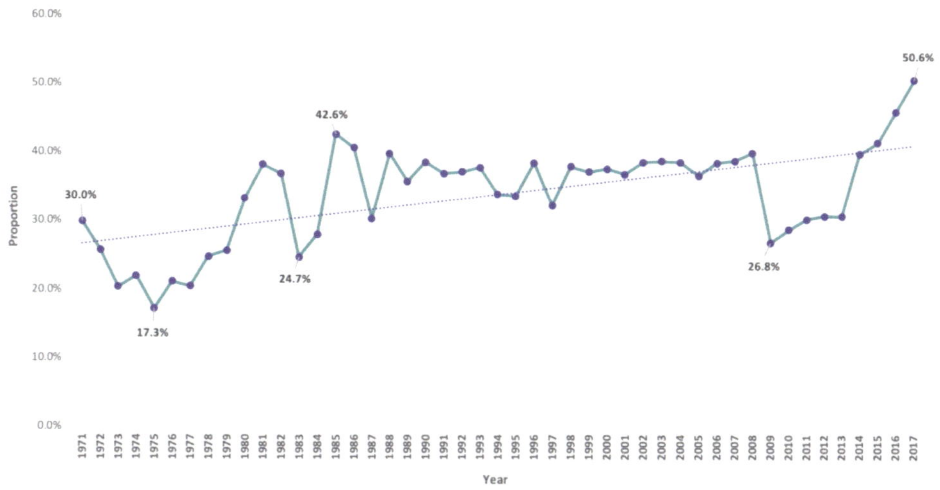

Figure 3.
Proportion of induced abortions in birth control surgery of family planning.

period of induced abortions is within 4 years after being married. Fourth, the proportion of repeat abortions is generally from 30 to 50%.

There are four main reasons related to the overall induced abortion in China [23–25], including unintended pregnancy with non-contraception, unintended pregnancy with contraception failure, sex selection (son preference especially in rural areas), and non-compliance with regulations of the family planning policies.

4. Relationship between the family planning policy and induced abortion in China

Since the founding of New China, the family planning policy is implemented chiefly relying on the means of contraception. Induced abortion is just a remedial measure for contraceptive failure. However, induced abortion was considered to have played an important role in the early period of the rapid decline of fertility rate after the implementation of the one-child policy in China, which attracted wide attention from the international community [26, 27].

The Chinese government has always advocated the contraceptive prevention for achieving the goal of birth control. The methods of intrauterine devices (IUD), sterilization, and tubal ligation were widely used in the early period of one-child policy. However, with the population boom in the late 1970s and the implementation of one-child policy in the early 1980s, the strict control indicator on fertility number has made induced abortion as one of the most important technical means for local governments at all levels in China from the 1980s to the early 1990s [28, 29], which resulted in the rapid increase of induced abortion rate and the rapid decline of fertility rate. Actually, at that time, the strict control indicator on fertility number, "one-vote negation system" of family planning, standard assessment on contraceptive rate, etc. had been the important ways for local government performance assessment and cadre promotion. What is more, many forced abortions have taken place in China [30, 31]. Since the mid-1990s, the family planning policy has undergone several adjustments and improvements, one important adjustment of which was the intervention action to reduce the number of policy-caused induced abortions, and followed by a significant decline of the induced abortion rate later in China [32].

The informed choice promoted in the International Conference on Population and Development in 1994 had provided good external environment for the transformation of China's contraceptive work, in particular, to reduce the induced abortion level [33]. Since March 1995, China began to implement the policy of informed choice and cancel part of related assessment indicators such as sterilization rate, induced abortion rate, etc. Through implementing the combined way, guided by the professional technical person and self-selection of contraceptive measures by the residents, it popularized the high-quality services of family planning and reduced the induced abortion rate [34]. The importance of the informed choice right was confirmed legally by the *Population and Family Planning Law of the People's Republic of China* promulgated in December 2001. Meanwhile, the legality of social upbringing fee or compensation fee was clarified for the first time, which made those women of unintended pregnancy have the possibility of unplanned fertility and further reduced the rate of induced abortion.

As one of the important assisted birth control methods in the implementation process of family planning policy in China, the level of induced abortion is significantly affected by the development trend of the family planning policy [7]. The rate of induced abortion when the one-child policy is implemented strictly to control the fertility rate is significantly higher than when the family planning policy is implemented moderately. A previous study showed that the induced abortion risk of married women of reproductive age was reduced by about 24% [32]. Under the background of moderate family planning policy, on the one hand, the establishment of social upbringing fee or compensation fee system makes it possible for women of reproductive age with unintended pregnancies to have the unplanned fertility choice; on the other hand, the implementation of informed choice policy gives women a certain amount of informed choice right in which they can choose the appropriate contraceptive measures by themselves, which can improve the contraception effect and avoid the unintended pregnancy to a certain extent, thus to reduce the risk of induced abortion relatively in China [35–39]. Using *China Population and Reproductive Health Survey Data* in 1997, Chen Wei analyzed the influencing factors of induced abortion of Chinese women, and the results showed that the family planning policy did not have significant impact on induced abortion of the women pregnant for the first time, but the effect would be increased significantly with the increase of pregnancy time [27, 40]. Other related studies found that unwanted pregnancy caused by contraceptive failure was the primary reason of induced abortion in China [26, 41]; however, non-compliance with the regulations of family planning policy was the main reason of induced abortion in rural areas in China [29].

In addition, although there is no clear regulation in the latest *Population and Family Planning Law of the People's Republic of China*, many local governments, family planning service institutions, and other related organizations have implemented the post-abortion family planning service (PAFPS) to reduce the risk of repeat abortion. Meanwhile, the *Family Planning Branch of Chinese Medical Association* has developed the guide of post-abortion family planning service [42].

5. Conclusions

In general, although induced abortion is never being regulated or clarified specifically in any related authoritative family planning policies or family planning laws actually in which it always emphasizes the importance of contraception, as the primary remedial measure of contraceptive failure, induced abortion has played a non-negligible and important role in controlling the fertility rate. Meanwhile, the induced abortion level in China is constantly changing with the development of family planning policy. Undeniably, China has achieved its objective of birth control by implementing the one-child policy, but it has also led to higher rate of induced abortion which means that Chinese women face higher risks of reproductive health. However, with the implementation of universal two-child policy and further advancement of PAFPS in China, the induced abortion level of family planning in China maybe further reduced which is worth looking forward to. Meanwhile, induced abortion of unmarried women who are not in the scope of family planning policy and service should be paid much more attention to. Therefore, although we cannot conclude that induced abortion is a part of family planning policy in China, it has been a part of the family planning service in China.

Acknowledgements

We appreciate the funding provided by the European Commission (EC)'s Seventh Framework Programme (FP7), grant number 282490.

Conflict of interest

We declare no conflict of interest.

Author details

Jinlin Liu[1], Yvon Englert[2] and Wei-Hong Zhang[2,3,4]*

1 Research Center for the Belt and Road Health Policy and Health Technology Assessment, Xi'an Jiaotong University, Xi'an, China

2 Research Laboratory for Human Reproduction, Faculty of Medicine, School of Public Health, Université Libre de Bruxelles (ULB), Brussels, Belgium

3 International Centre for Reproductive Health (ICRH), Department of Public Health and Primary Care, Ghent University, Ghent, Belgium

4 Research Centre for Public Health, Tsinghua University, Beijing, China

*Address all correspondence to: weihong.zhang@ugent.be

References

[1] Liu H. Family planning has existed since ancient times. Culture and History Vision. 2012;**10**:56-57

[2] Zhang Y et al. Modern Talent. 2013;**6**:46-47

[3] Dou D. The implementation of family planning in ancient China. Decision & Information. 2014;**4**:58-59

[4] Zhang Y. Encourage fertility: The family planning policy in ancient China. Culture and History Vision. 2014;**6**:59-60

[5] Wang C. History of the Chinese family planning program: 1970-2010. Contraception. 2012;**85**:563-569

[6] Guo Z. The population thought of Mao Zedong and the reconsideration on family planning policy of China in the 1950s and 1960s. Northwest Population Journal. 2003;(4):2-7

[7] Zheng X, Pang L, Tellier S, et al. The changing patterns of abortion among married women in China, 1984-2005. European Journal of Obstetrics, Gynecology, and Reproductive Biology. 2013;**166**:70-75

[8] Yu X. Review and comment on the thirty years' family planning policy in China. China Population Today. 2008;**25**(5):31-34

[9] Wu C, Xie N. Review and outlook on the thirty years' population policy in China from 1980 to 2010. Gansu Social Sciences. 2011;**1**:1-5

[10] Qiao X. Evolution of the family planning policy in China. Russian Central Asian & East European Market. 2016;**3**:19-24

[11] Ruo Z. From beginning to end of the family planning policy's publishment in China. Wan Qing. 2015;**12**:50-55

[12] National Health and Family Planning Commission of the People's Republic of China. China Health and Family Planning Statistics 2015. Pecking Beijing: Union Medical College Press; 2015

[13] Zhou L. The family planning policy in China: Effects, limitations and future. Journal of Harbin University. 2014;**35**(7):34-37

[14] Fu T. Discussion on the reason of abortion sin's law transplantation's failure in modern China. Journal of Heilongjiang Administrative Cadre Institute of Politics and Law. 2015;**5**:30-33

[15] Tian Y, Jiao P. Brief textual research on abortion in ancient China. The Journal of Medicine and Philosophy. 2007;**28**(5):64-65

[16] Tang H. Crime and non-crime: Abortion of China in the 20th century. Jianghan Tribune. 2011;**9**:128-131

[17] Ma S, Yu Q. Analysis on the criminal law and eugenics and healthcare law in Taiwan: From the research perspective of abortion behavior. Jingyue Journal. 2013;**1**:99-103

[18] Cheng Y, Xu X, Xu J, et al. The need for integrating family planning and post-abortion care in China. International Journal of Gynecology & Obstetrics. 2008;**103**(2):140-143

[19] Cheng Y, Guo X, Li Y, et al. Repeat induced abortions and contraceptive practices among unmarried young women seeking an abortion in China. International Journal of Gynecology & Obstetrics. 2004;**87**(2):199-202

[20] Cheng Y, Ren S. Analysis on situation, problems and solutions on the induced abortion service in China. Chinese Journal of Family Planning & Gynecotokology. 2011;**3**(5):5-8

[21] Chen Q. Research progress on the induced abortion and contraception in China. Chinese and Foreign Women Health. 2011;**19**(4):124-125

[22] Wang H, Long L, Cai H, et al. Contraception and unintended pregnancy among unmarried female university students: A cross-sectional study from China. PLoS One. 2015;**10**(6):e0130212

[23] Wang D, Yan H, Feng Z. Abortion as a backup method for contraceptive failure in China. Journal of Biosocial Science. 2004;**36**(03):279-287

[24] Li H, Li DQ, Li HQ, et al. Contraception and induced abortions for women of reproductive age married in recent years in rural areas of Shandong, China. Gynecologic and Obstetric Investigation. 2009;**68**(3):174-180

[25] Lancet T. Sex imbalance in China. The Lancet. 2011;**378**(9793):742

[26] Wang Y, Becker S, Chow LP, et al. Induced abortion in eight provinces of China. Asia-Pacific Journal of Public Health. 1991;**5**(1):32-40

[27] Chen W, Zhuang Y. Analysis on determinants of provincial-level induced abortion in China. Population Journal. 2004;**3**:16-21

[28] Feng Z, Chen H, Charles C. Induced abortion in Xian City, China. International Family Planning Perspectives. 1983;**9**(3):81-85

[29] Qiao X. Analysis on women induced abortion situation in China. Journal of Population Research. 2002;**26**(3):16-25

[30] Watts J. Chinese officials accused of forcing abortions in Shandong. Lancet. 2005;**366**(9493):1253

[31] Li Y. Reflections on the causes of forced abortion in China. Lancet. 2012;**380**(9844):804

[32] Wang C. A sociological empirical research on induced abortion in China: 1979-2012. Social Sciences in China. 2014;**10**:62-78

[33] Chen G, Pang L, Zheng X. Analysis on situation, trend and influence factors of the induced abortion in China. Chinese Journal of Population Science. 2007;**5**:49-59

[34] Zhang E, Gu B, Xie Z. Evaluation Reports on High-Quality Service in the First Batch of Pilot Counties of the National Family Planning Commission. Beijing: China Population Publishing House; 1999

[35] Li Y, Wu Y, Sun Z, et al. Analysis on the impact of improving family planning service quality on reducing the induced abortion. Journal of Reproduction and Contraception. 1999;**6**:357-362

[36] Wu J, Li Y, Chen X, et al. The effect of community intervention of informed choice on contraception behavior of the rural married women of childbearing age. Fudan University Journal of Medical Sciences. 2006;**33**(3):332-335

[37] Wang C. The effects of the client-centered police of informed choice of contraceptives for induced abortion in China. Population and Development. 2010;**16**(3):17-26+112

[38] Wang C. A test of the impacts of the client-centered contraceptive policy of informed choice on induced abortion in China. South China Population. 2011;**26**(1):7-13

[39] Wang C. An evaluation of the effects of the client-centered contraceptive policy of informed choice by fixed effect modeling: the cases analysis of the changes in the married reproductive-age individuals' contraceptive measures taken. South China Population. 2012;**27**(2):1-6

[40] Chen W. Determinants of induced abortion in China: A multilevel

analysis. Market Demographic Analysis. 2002;**8**(5):11-20

[41] Wang D, Diamond I. The impact on fertility of contraceptive failure in China in the 1980s. Journal of Biosocial Science. 1995;**27**(03):277-284

[42] Family planning branch of Chinese Medical Association. Post-abortion family planning service guide. Chinese Journal of Obstetrics and Gynecology. 2011;**46**(4):319-320

Chapter 3

East-West Divide in Abortion Behaviour in the EU Countries Since 1990: Ongoing or Vanished Differentiation?

Jiřina Kocourková

Abstract

In the late 1980s, the East-West divide by birth control was identified in Europe as both parts differed by contraceptive practices and abortion rates. The aim of this chapter is to investigate changes in abortion behaviour and 'whether the East-West divide in abortion behaviour remained relevant by 2009'. As the large variation in terms of abortion rates and contraceptive patterns is still identified in Europe, we want to investigate 'to what extent it has reflected in the birth control patterns'. The main results could be summed up as follows: (1) the East-West divide in abortion behaviour was distorted, but not fully eliminated. Besides the former Eastern and Western abortion patterns, the new 'low abortion' pattern has emerged. (2) Within the EU countries, convergent trends towards lower abortion level were identified since 1990. However, as regards the structure of abortions, a pattern of divergence has been apparent due to differences in transition to modern contraception use. (3) The use of modern methods of contraception rather depends on structural macro-level factors and contextual incentives and barriers as the impact of individual characteristics on the use of contraception does not differ much between countries under study.

Keywords: abortion, contraception, abortion rate, fertility, East-West division

1. Introduction

In the late 1980s, the East-West divide by birth control was identified in Europe as both parts differed by contraceptive practices and abortion rates [1]. This East-West divide resulted from divergent historical trends between the two regions [2]. 'Abortion culture' was the term used to characterise the nature of birth regulating behaviour in the formerly socialist countries of Soviet bloc, that is, Eastern Europe, up to the end of the 1980s [3, 4]. Liberal abortion legislation made induced abortions easily accessible as well as socially acceptable. Abortions were highly prevalent because they were available upon request and mostly free of charge [5]. Due to its wide availability, easy accessibility and social acceptability, abortion became an element of reproductive culture with moral legitimacy [6]. In most countries, women had an average of one to two lifetime abortions. In Soviet Union and Romania, however, women with three to five abortions were not uncommon [7, 8].

Modern contraceptives (hormonal contraception) were less available and of poor quality; thus, most couples relied on traditional methods [4].

On the contrary, in Western Europe, modern contraceptives were widely available, and registered abortion rates in Western European countries were significantly lower than those in Eastern European countries [8]. One of the explanations of such profound differences in birth control practices lays in different timing of liberalization of abortion law in Western and Eastern European countries. In most former socialist countries of Eastern Europe, abortion law was liberalised in 1950s and predated the spread of hormonal contraception since the late 1960s. In most Western European countries abortion law was liberalised later, in the 1970s and 1980s, thus after the spread of modern contraceptives [9]. In Western Europe, the transition towards the dominant use of modern contraception was termed the contraceptive revolution [10] and took place during the 1960s and 1970s [8].

Moreover, abortion played different roles in these two regions as women who had abortions differed sharply between the countries of Eastern and Western Europe [1]. In the Eastern European countries, abortion was used to limit family size once certain parity had been reached; thus induced abortion was the most frequently requested by married women with two or more children. The highest abortion rates were registered in women in their late 20s and 30s and formed a rather 'late abortion pattern' [4]. On the other hand, in Western European countries, abortion was used primarily in case of mistimed pregnancies, so most women who had abortions were young, childless and unmarried [1]. The highest abortion rates were the most typical for young age categories of women, thus formed a pattern that could be labelled as 'early abortion pattern'.

Before 1990, the East-West differences in Europe were apparent not only in birth control methods but also in fertility patterns. In Western Europe, large-scale changes in childbearing were under way since the 1970s. Modern contraceptives were instrumental in childbearing postponement to the later age of women and fertility decline below replacement level in this region [11]. In contrast, in Eastern Europe, the early childbearing pattern characterised by the highest fertility rates of women in the age of 20–24 years and fertility around replacement level was kept in the Eastern Europe until the beginning of the 1990s [12]. Accordingly, the early childbearing pattern and late abortion pattern were closely connected. Besides, since the contraceptive prevalence was low, trends in fertility and abortion rates were inversely related [13].

At the beginning of the 1990s, the East-West divide was characterised by the profound difference in both the abortion level and the contraceptive prevalence. While in Western and Northern Europe, the abortion rate varied between 14 and 22 abortions per 1000 women aged 15–44; in Eastern Europe, it was on average 88 per 1000 [14]. As regards the contraceptive use in Western and Northern Europe, more than 94% of users employed modern effective methods (pills, IUD, and barrier methods) in contrast to only 44% of them in Eastern Europe [8]. Since 1990, political and socio-economic transformation has occurred in Eastern Europe that also reflected in profound changes of the reproductive behaviour. The early childbearing pattern gradually vanished as a result of transition towards later childbearing. In Eastern Europe, decrease in both fertility and abortion rates was registered in the 1990s [12]. Trends in fertility and abortion rates ceased to be inversely related and became independent in some countries [15]. Although contraceptive use increased and abortion rate steadily decreased in most Eastern European countries during last decades, in some countries, abortion rates remain relatively high (42 per 1000 in 2010–2014), more than 20% of women in reproductive age still relied on traditional methods and the level of unmet need for contraception varied between 15 and 20% [16].

The 1990s are regarded as the period of major discontinuities and a growing differentiation in Eastern Europe. Although there were some studies on abortion trends since 1990, most of them related to comparison across world regions with no specific attention to Western or Eastern European countries [17–19]. Nevertheless, more attention was paid to European cross-national comparisons in contraceptive practices [20–23]. Recently, two studies supported the continuation of East-West divide in contraceptive use [16, 24]; however, in these two studies, the continuation of East-West divide was taken as presumption to be confirmed, and the increased regional variation, particularly within Eastern Europe, was ignored.

Furthermore, less attention has also been devoted to assessment of changes in abortion in relation to changes in contraceptive use in Eastern Europe despite investigation of the relationship between trends in contraceptive use and in the incidence of induced abortion has been a subject of many studies on other world regions [25–27]. Interestingly, findings have not been consistent as increased contraceptive use need not necessarily lead to lower abortion rates and vice versa [26]. Fertility change plays the key role of mediating factor, which means that in case of a rapid fertility decline significant decrease in abortion need not occur as only increased contraceptive use by itself may be unable to meet the growing need for fertility regulation. This was particularly relevant for Eastern Europe in the 1990s.

In the 2000s, widening of EU and further integration of Europe were expected to contribute also to demographic convergence within EU. Many countries in Eastern Europe took steps towards reforming their reproductive health policies and programmes related to family planning as well as discussed the factors that could promote increased contraceptive use and decline in reliance on abortion [28]. The aim of this chapter is to investigate changes in abortion behaviour and 'whether the East-West divide in abortion behaviour remained relevant by 2009'. As the large variation in terms of abortion rates [14] and contraceptive patterns [24] is still identified in Europe, we want to investigate 'to what extent it has reflected in the birth control patterns'. Has the former East-West divide remained or has the new one emerged? 2009 was taken for detailed analysis of the relationship between abortion and contraceptive behaviour in EU countries as the most detailed data on abortion and, in particular, on contraceptive use were available'.

2. Data and methods

Data sources on abortion and birth control method are of different quality; therefore, several international data sources were used. The international databases referred on abortions included Eurostat and [29]. As regards the contraception use, data collected by the UN [30] and data from [29] were relevant. Moreover, data from the Generation and Gender Survey, the second wave, (2007–2008; [31]) were used for detailed analysis of characteristics of users. Furthermore, cross-country differences in abortion legislation should be taken into account when making a comparison. Only 21 out of 28 EU countries with liberal legislation and available data on abortions were considered for analysis. Ireland, Malta, and Poland were not included into analysis due to restrictive legislation [29]. Austria, Croatia, Cyprus, and Luxembourg were not included as no national or international data on abortions were available. The time limit for an induced abortion is not uniform across countries [29]. It is 10–14 weeks of gestation in most EU Member States, but higher in Sweden (18 weeks) and the UK (24 weeks). Countries have also different policies and practices with regard to the time limit for induced abortion for a foetal or maternal indication. Parental authorization for induced abortion of women under the age of

18 years is required in 11 countries under study: Czech Republic, Denmark, Estonia, Greece, Hungary, Italy, Latvia, Lithuania, Portugal, Sweden, and Slovakia. Finally, completeness of available data, defined as covering at least 90% of all legal abortions [17], was reported for 10 countries from Western Europe (Belgium, Denmark, Finland, France, Germany, Italy, Portugal, the Netherlands, Sweden, and the United Kingdom) and for 6 countries from Eastern Europe (Bulgaria, Czech Republic, Estonia, Hungary, Slovakia, and Slovenia). Higher risk of under-reporting could be found in Latvia, Lithuania, and Romania, and also in Greece and Spain. It relates particularly to abortions performed in private clinics or abortions among migrants. Some national statistics may not include medical abortions. By 2010, medical abortion was not allowed in five Eastern European countries under study: Czech Republic, Hungary, Lithuania, Romania, and Slovakia.

Comparative analysis included both the changes in the level and structure of induced abortions, and changes in contraceptive practice. General abortion rate is defined as the number of legally induced abortion per 1000 women aged 15–49. Age-specific induced abortion rate is defined as the number of induced abortion of women per 1000 women of given age group. Contraceptive prevalence rate is defined as the percentage of women in reproductive age (15–49 years) or their partners who were using a contraceptive method at a particular point in time [30]. The analysis of relationship between contraception and abortion was based on data that were obtained for 18 European countries from online databases of Eurostat as regards abortions and from the UN [30] as regards prevalence of modern contraceptive use (percentage using contraception among women who are married or in a union, modern method: sterilization, pills, injectable, implant, IUD, male condom, or vaginal barrier method). Cluster analysis of birth control indicators was used to give more detailed insight into current typology of abortion behaviour in the EU. The following four indicators were included into cluster analysis: general abortion rate in 2009, abortion rate of women aged 15–19 years in 2009, ratio of abortion rates of women in the age group 20–24 to 25–29 years in 2009, and contraceptive prevalence rate of modern methods (latest available data). These indicators were selected to capture the specific aspect of abortion behaviour that could differentiate between abortion patterns. Greece, Portugal, and the Netherlands were not included in cluster analysis as abortions by age group of women were not available for these countries.

Finally, data from the second wave of Generation and Gender Survey [31] were analysed as they provide more information about contraceptive behaviour in selected three countries: the Czech Republic (2008), France (2008), and Bulgaria (2007). This survey collected representative data from people aged between 18 and 79 in European countries. The key feature of the survey is the cross-national comparability by providing the survey design, a standard questionnaire, and common definitions and instructions in all countries [32, 33]. The core question, investigating current use of contraceptive methods, was 'Are you doing or using anything to prevent pregnancy?'. For the purpose of comparison, only data concerning women of reproductive age (18–44) were included in the analysis. Furthermore, the analysis was restricted to women of reproductive age, who had a partner—whether cohabiting or not—at the time of the interview. Therefore, the total number of women aged 18–44, eligible for analysis, was 1522 in the Czech Republic, 1334 in France, and 556 in Bulgaria. We utilised SPSS version 20 to analyse the data and, more specifically, to compare the percentage distributions of female respondents by contraceptive status. In the event that respondents reported multiple contraceptive methods, only the most effective method was taken into account. The traditional and less effective methods cited in the analysis included withdrawal and periodic abstinence. The pills, IUDs, and condoms were all considered to be effective contraceptives. However, when applying multivariate statistical analysis to identify differences in the use of modern contraceptives by individual characteristics, only the pills and IUDs were included into calculations. Adjusted odds ratios were used to assess predictors for the use of the modern contraceptives. We applied binary logistic regression to adjust for potential confounding factors. Age, type of partnership, number of children, and education were included as independent variables, while the use or non-use of pill or IUD was the dependent binary variable.

3. Results

Changes in cross-national variations in abortion rate can be assessed when plotting EU countries according to both values in 1989 and 2009 (**Figure 1**). Interestingly, a group of Eastern European countries could be clearly separated from Western European countries, which suggests continuation of East-West divide. It is apparent that Eastern European countries differed from the West region by both level of abortion rates and by abortion trends between 1989 and 2009. As all Eastern European countries registered a profound decline in abortion rates during this period, variations in abortion rate across the East region were significantly reduced. While the general abortion rate in 1989 ranged between 35 (Slovenia) and 66 (Bulgaria and Estonia) abortions per 1000 women aged 15–49, in 2009, it was only between 7.7 (Slovakia) and 25 (Estonia) abortions per 1000 women aged 15–49. Interestingly, the abortion rate fell most precipitously in Slovakia and the Czech Republic, i.e. in those countries that did not register the highest incidence of abortion. In most of the countries, the decline in abortion rate occurred predominantly in the 1990s, and after 2003, the pace of the decrease slowed down [17].

In contrast to the East region, variation in abortion rates within the West region in 1989 was not large as Western European countries mostly registered low abortion rates, between 3 (Greece) and 14 (France) abortions per 1000 women aged 15–49 (**Figure 1**). Furthermore, although abortion rates held fairly steady in Finland and

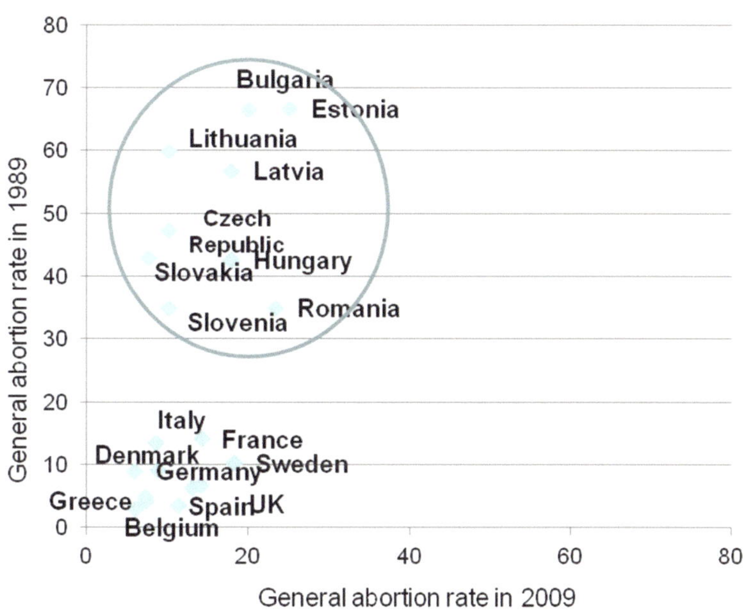

Figure 1.
EU countries by general abortion rates in 1989 and 2009 (abortions per 1000 women aged 15–49).

France, and Italy together with Germany registered decline in the abortion rate, the dominant trend in this region was an increase in abortion rate. It regarded both countries with rather higher abortion rate within this region, that is, Sweden, the UK, Denmark, and those with low abortion rate, that is, Greece, Spain, Belgium, and the Netherlands. The steepest rise (from 3 to 11 abortions per 100 women) was registered in Spain, which was attributed to the rapidly growing immigrant population. Similarly, immigration is behind the increase in abortions also in other countries. Recent studies indicated that 25–36% of abortions in Finland, the Netherlands, and Sweden were requested from foreign-born women, largely those of non-European origin [17].

Contrary to previous findings, ordering of countries according to abortion rates in 2009 rather suggests vanishing of the former East-West divide (**Figure 2**). Although the highest abortion rates were found in Eastern European countries (Estonia, Romania, and Bulgaria) and the lowest abortion rates were found in Western European countries (Germany, Greece, the Netherlands, Portugal, and Belgium), Slovakia together with Czech Republic, Slovenia, and Lithuania reached levels even lower than those registered in five countries of the former West region, that is, Sweden, France, the UK, Denmark, and Spain. Thus, as regards the abortion rate in 2009, a group of four countries that were formerly a part of Eastern Europe no longer belonged to the East region.

Cluster analysis based on birth control indicators of 18 EU countries in 2009 revealed the existence of three clusters of countries that differ by both level and structure of abortion as well as by contraceptive prevalence rate of modern method (**Figure 3**). These clusters are characterised by differences in average values of general abortion rate, abortion rate of teenage women, ratio of abortion rate of women aged 20–24 and 25–29, and contraceptive prevalence rate of modern method (**Table 1**). The first cluster can be taken as a continuation of the former 'early abortion pattern' as it consisted predominantly of Western and Northern European countries, Denmark, Sweden, Finland, the UK, and France. Newly, Hungary and Spain emerged in this cluster. As the ratio of abortion rate in age 20–24 to 25–29 is higher than 1, the concentration of abortions mainly among young women is the main characteristic of this cluster. Moreover, the abortion rate of teenage women is quite high despite the high contraceptive prevalence of modern methods in these

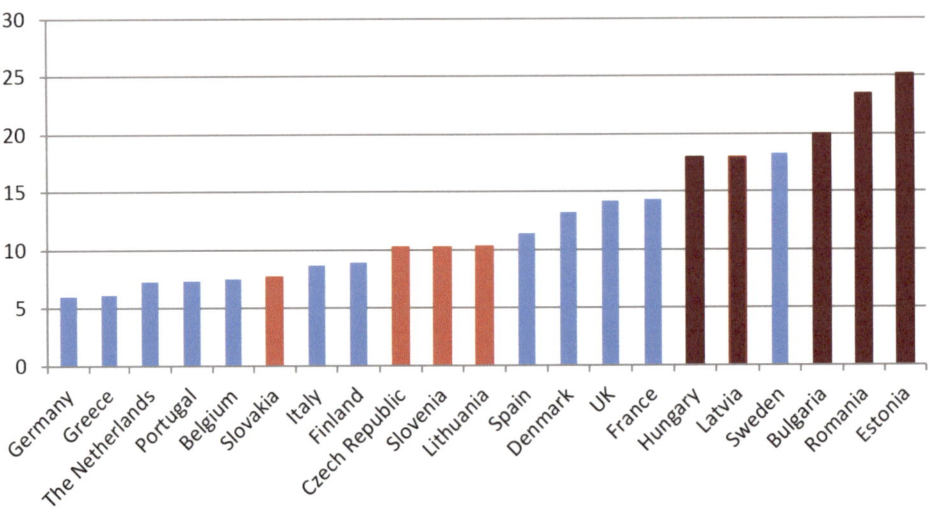

Figure 2.
General abortion rate in 2009 in EU Member States (abortions per 1000 women aged 15–49).

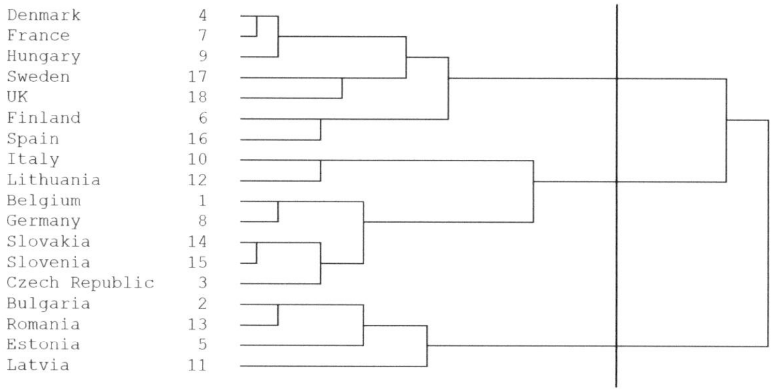

Figure 3.
Dendrogram with three clusters of EU countries determined by similarities in abortion pattern in 2009. Notes: Cluster analysis using average linkage between groups, SPSS version 20. Variables included into cluster analysis: abortions per 1000 women aged 15–49, abortions per 1000 women aged 15–19, ratio of abortion rates in 20–24 to 25–29 (2009), and contraceptive prevalence rate of modern methods.

Cluster	Pattern	Countries	Abortions per 1000 women aged 15–49	Abortion rate in age 15–19	Ratio of abortion rate in age 20–24 to 25–29	Contraceptive prevalence of modern methods %
First	Early abortion	Denmark, France, Hungary, Sweden, the UK, Finland, Spain	13-Mar	16.53	Jan-16	64.3
Second	High abortion	Bulgaria, Romania, Estonia, Latvia	21.63	16.93	0.95	47.43
Third	Low abortion	Italy, Lithuania, Belgium, Germany, Slovakia, Slovenia, Czech Republic	Aug-32	Jul-30	1.00	69.10

Table 1.
Distribution of 18 EU countries into three clusters, the average values of indicators.

countries. The abortion rate of teenage women is even as high as in the second cluster of countries characterised by 'high abortion pattern' typical for Bulgaria, Romania, Estonia, and Latvia, that is, the Eastern European countries. Abortion rate was reduced in these countries; however, it was still high in all age groups in comparison with other EU countries. Ratio of abortion rate in age 20–24 to 25–29 is only slightly lower than 1 suggesting that dominant characteristics became the relatively high abortion level instead of highest frequency of abortions among women in the late 20s and early 30s as it was two decades before. The third 'low abortion' cluster emerged as a new one and consists of a mix of countries, that is, Italy, Belgium, Germany, and four Eastern European countries that are part of the East region: Lithuania, Slovenia,

Slovakia, and the Czech Republic. These countries have low abortion rate combined with high contraceptive prevalence of modern methods in common.

Looking at those clusters in more detail, three patterns of abortion behaviour in EU countries can be better identified (**Figure 4**). France was selected from the first cluster as representative of the former Western 'early abortion pattern' characterised by high abortion rate among women younger than 25 years and particularly among teenage women. Although in France the highest percentage of women using pills was found (**Figure 5**), it is connected with the highest propensity to end an unwanted pregnancy among teenage woman, suggesting the increase in demand for fertility control due to a delay in fertility has not been sufficiently met yet. Bulgaria was selected from the second cluster as the representative of the 'high abortion pattern' (**Figure 4**). Women aged 20–29 years accounted for the highest frequency of abortions, and the abortion rate of women aged 30–34 is also considerably high. Interestingly, the abortion rate of youngest Bulgarian women aged 15–19 is comparable with that of French women in this age group. Behind the high abortion rate are the low improvements in modern contraceptive practice, as only 40% of Bulgarian women of reproductive age use modern methods of birth control (**Figure 5**). While these two clusters confirm the continuation of the former 'Western' and 'Eastern' patterns, the third one has emerged recently as a result of a rapid increased use of effective contraceptive methods. The Czech Republic could be taken as a representative of this 'low abortion pattern', with high contraceptive prevalence of modern methods (78%) and low general abortion rate (12%). The fall in abortion rates was most pronounced in the age group with traditionally highest rates of abortion, that is, between 20 and 34 years, which resulted in diminishing the differences in abortion rates between all age groups.

The comparison of contraceptive behaviour in the Czech Republic, France, and Bulgaria based on data from the second wave of the Generation and Gender Survey highlights differences in family planning practice in the three countries. While both in the Czech Republic and France the highest percentage of women aged 18–44 years and having partner uses the pills (45% and 49%), in Bulgaria, the dominant effective method of contraception is condom (23%). In contrast to the Czech Republic and France, 20% of Bulgarian women aged 18–44 years and having partner rely on traditional and less-effective method. Furthermore, in

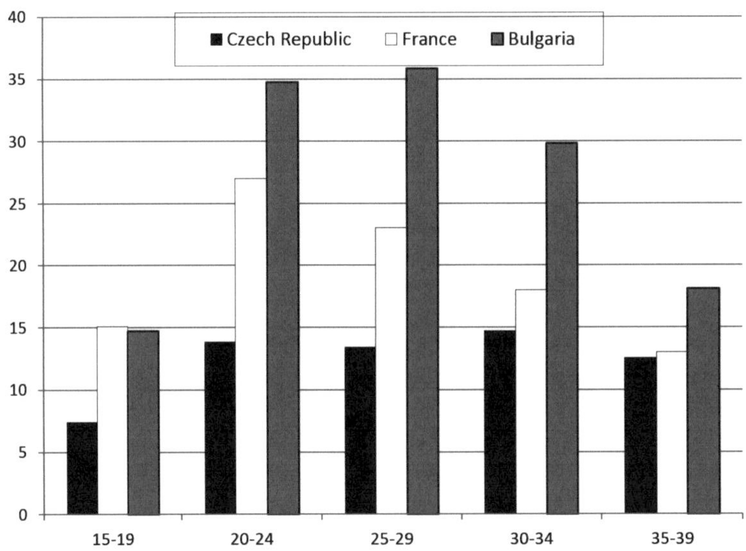

Figure 4.
Age-specific abortion rates in 2009 (abortions per 1000 women).

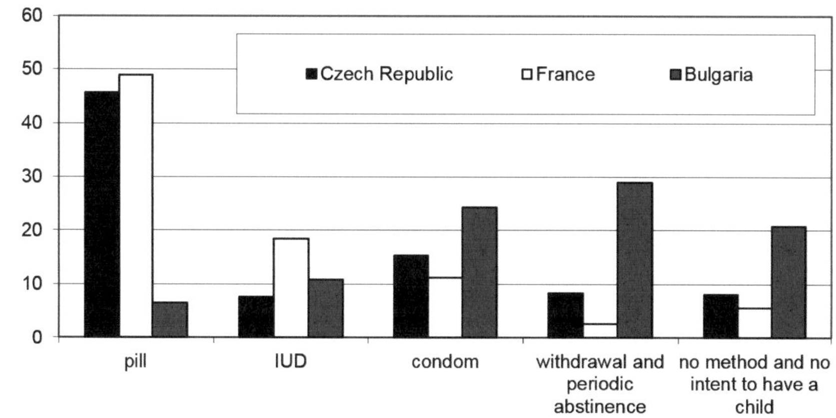

Figure 5.
Percentage distribution of women by method of contraception, generation and gender survey, second wave, and women aged 18–44 having a partner. Data source: GGS2 (second wave), Czech Republic (2008), France (2008), and Bulgaria (2007).

	Czech Republic	France	Bulgaria
Type of partnership			
Living together (ref.)	1	1	1
Not living together	1.78^{***}	1.43^{**}	1.35^{**}
Age group			
18–24	8.00^{***}	6.65^{***}	3.69^{***}
25–29	2.83^{***}	3.37^{***}	2.23^{***}
30–34	1.85^{***}	1.93^{**}	1.45^{**}
35–39	1.34^{**}	1.45^{**}	1.14^{*}
40–44 (ref.)	1	1	1
Number of children			
0 (ref.)	1	1	1
1	1.02	1.12	1.15
2	1.20	1.23	1.11
3 +	1.09	1.13	1.21
Educational level			
Lower (ref.)	1	1	1
Secondary	1.06	1.31^{*}	1.12
Higher	1.26^{*}	1.42^{*}	1.39^{**}
Number of users	1522	1334	556

Data source: GGS2 (second wave), Czech Republic (2008), France (2008), Bulgaria (2007).
Note: Binary logistic regression, $^{***}p < 0.01$; $^{**}p < 0.05$; $^{*}p < 0.1$, *SPSS version 20.*

Table 2.
Determinants of contraceptive use of the pill or IUD by women in selected countries (odds ratio).

Bulgaria, high level of unmet need for contraception probably exists as almost 20% of Bulgarian women do not practice fertility control although they do not intend to have a child. Other studies also confirmed the highest prevalence of non-use and traditional method use [16, 28]. The impact of individual characteristics on the use of modern method (pills and IUD) was analysed by binary logistic regression. After adjustment for all characteristics in **Table 2**, the use of the pill was found significantly associated with the type of partnership, age, and education in all three countries. The Czech youngest women are eight times more likely to use the pill or IUD than women aged 40–44 years old while Bulgarian youngest women less than four times. Not living with a partner significantly predicts the use of the pill as well as higher education attainment. Interestingly, the number of children did not prove to be a statistically significant predictor in all countries under study.

4. Discussion

Between 1989 and 2009, a sharp decrease in abortion rates in Eastern Europe narrowed variations in abortion behaviour across EU countries. We have found that the East-West divide in abortion behaviour was distorted, but not fully eliminated. Up to 2009, the main differentiating signs remained similar to the former abortion patterns as high abortion rates across all age group of women were still typical for the 'Eastern' abortion pattern and the high abortion rate of young women kept to be typical for the 'Western' abortion pattern. However, a considerable decline in the abortion rate in some Eastern European countries (Lithuania, Slovakia, the Czech Republic, and Slovenia) resulted in formation of a new abortion pattern different from the former Eastern and Western patterns. These countries joined some Western European countries that also registered a decline of already low abortion rate (Italy and Germany).

However, during the period under study, Eastern European countries started to differ not only in abortion behaviour but also in contraceptive practice. Some recent cross-country studies disregard that Eastern European countries significantly differed by the increase in the use of modern contraceptives since 1990. The study of Dereuddre et al. [16, 24] confirmed that the East-West divide in contraceptive use continued to be relevant up until recently. Accordingly, Western European countries were characterised by the widespread use of modern contraception, and Central and Eastern European countries were characterised by a high prevalence of traditional methods. However, this study did not recognise that in some Eastern European countries, in particular the Czech Republic and Slovakia, the transition to the dominant use of modern contraceptives occurred in such profound way that it could be considered as complete [13, 15]. Rapid transition to use of modern contraceptive method prevented a shift of high abortion rate to the youngest age group of women similarly to the characteristics of the former 'West' abortion pattern. Instead, a new pattern of low abortion across all age group could be formed.

Thus, around 2009, three abortion patterns could be determined. The 'early abortion pattern' continued to exist although it was no more dominant only for Northwestern part of Europe as Spain and Hungary showed similar characteristics. The relatively high teenage abortion rate and abortion rate of women aged 20–24 years is due to the great variation in quality and quantity of sexuality education and sexual and reproductive health services financing, and partly due to a growing demand for abortion from women in ethnic minority groups [29]. Moreover, the longer gestational limit for an induced abortion in some countries (the UK and Sweden) could also contribute to the maintenance of this model. France was taken as a typical example of this abortion pattern. Despite abortion rates remain stable in France since the early 1990s, the age of the women who have abortions decreased during this period [19]. Since the mid-1990s, abortion rates below the age of 25 years increased while remaining stable at other ages. It seems that this early abortion pattern was even strengthened in the context of delayed childbearing. Besides, the extension of gestational limit in 2001 and legalization of medical abortion in private practices in 2004 and in family-planning centres in 2009 probably also contributed to fixing this pattern in France.

Interestingly, the other two countries came out to belong to this 'early abortion pattern'. Spain was the country where the abortion rate has significantly increased in the 2000s. It was probably due to an increase in immigrant population as immigrant women's abortion rate was found three times higher than that of Spanish women [33]. Similar findings relate also to other countries with a higher proportion of immigrant populations like Sweden and Finland since immigrants have greater difficulties to access contraception. Finally, in Hungary, improvements in contraceptive use were registered as the pill became the most frequently used contraceptive methods instead of barrier methods [34]. However, the increase in contraceptive prevalence did not prevent unintended pregnancies of young women since the abortion rate among young women remained relatively high.

The 'late abortion pattern' typical for Eastern European countries prior to 1990 seems to have been transformed to 'high abortion pattern' for part of these countries. Thus, the specific Eastern European pattern continues to exist in the context of more liberal abortion law than prior to 1990. This pattern is not characterised by high abortion rate dominantly in older age of women like prior to 1990 when most of abortion law enabled women to request an abortion only after having a certain number of children. Despite a decline in abortion level and an increase in contraceptive prevalence by 2009, these countries continued to differ from the rest of EU countries by higher abortion rate across the whole reproductive age of women. The increase in contraceptive prevalence itself was not a sufficient determinant of reduction of abortions in any age group as mainly the increase in use of less effective methods occurred. Rather the shift in method mix towards modern contraception could induce the more profound decline in abortion level [26]. Abortion rate is high in societies where low contraceptive prevalence or use of ineffective methods is combined with low-fertility norms, and in societies with a high propensity to rely on induced abortion [25]. Accordingly, some increase in contraception prevalence was probably not accompanied by the replacement of traditional methods with more effective alternatives in these countries. Accordingly, the high abortion rate still registered in Bulgaria, Estonia, Latvia, and Romania in 2009 can be explained by high prevalence of using traditional method and still high propensity to rely on induced abortion despite sexual and reproductive health programmes were established in the 1990s [28]. Only modern contraception can replace abortion. The previous studies [26] showed the inverse of the relationship when the proportion of women using traditional methods was plotted against abortion rate, that is, reliance on abortion was increasing with the prevalence of traditional method of contraception.

Besides, fertility decline that occurred in Romania in the first half of the 1990s was not sufficiently compensated by contraceptive prevalence rise and resulted even in the temporal increase in abortion rate [35]). Furthermore, this fertility decline related to the births of second and third-order and it did not contribute to first birth postponement [36]. Although subsequent decline in abortion rate has been registered, some experts pointed out that the number of unreported, privately performed induced abortions particularly in Romania has increased substantially [17]. The declines rather represent a combination of real declines in incidence and a shift to unreported abortions. Significant reduction in the abortion rate would be obtained if most traditional contraceptive methods shifted to modern methods. Decline in abortion rate without the widespread use of effective birth control methods is not sufficient to encourage the shift in reproduction pattern. Van de Kaa [11] identified modern contraceptives as the means that made possible not only the low fertility but they also acted as a catalyst of changes in reproductive pattern within the concept of second demographic transition.

On the contrary, other four Eastern European countries, the Czech Republic, Lithuania, Slovakia, and Slovenia, that formerly registered high abortion rate, contributed to form the new 'low abortion pattern' characterised by low abortion rates across all age group of women. This pattern is based on the increased use of efficient modern contraceptive methods and could be also found in Italy, Belgium, and Germany. During the 1990s, fertility decline occurred in the Czech Republic, Lithuania, Slovakia, and Slovenia and did not result in any an increase in unmet need for family planning as no increase in abortion rate was observed. Instead, a decline in abortion in all age group of women was registered. Both young and older women improved their contraceptive behaviour although the highest increase in use of the pill was registered among young women below the age of 25 years. As a result, young women do not rely on abortion when planning childbearing but rather prevent unintended pregnancy. So once there were conditions for effective family planning, the abortion rate could rapidly fall without any legislative restrictions on access to abortions [15]. The increase in contraceptive use has been sufficient to encompass both the sharp decline in abortion and the trend towards fertility postponement. The spread of modern contraceptive methods facilitates fertility changes and may result in altering norms regarding fertility regulation, but also in reverse, attitudes with regard to contraceptive use may be shifted [11]. Accordingly, significant improvements in contraceptive practice in these Eastern European countries might encourage shaping of a new reproduction pattern, that is, late fertility pattern, as it was documented in the Czech Republic [13].

Analysis of the link between contraceptive use of modern methods and individual characteristics has brought findings that are consistent with other studies, in particular as regards the educational attainment [16, 23, 24, 37]. Our results also confirmed that highly educated women are more likely to use modern contraception in all analysed countries across all abortion patterns. Moreover, young women are the most receptive to use hormonal contraceptives. While the proportions of users of contraceptive methods vary considerably particularly between the Czech Republic and France on one side and Bulgaria on the other, the characteristics of the users of modern effective methods were found to be similar. Therefore, the causes of these variations might be partly explained by the macro-level factors [38]. Variations observed in contraceptive prevalence and in the mix of methods are determined both by the socio-demographic characteristics of the respondents and by macro-level factors such as legislation, reproductive health care system, family planning programme, or cultural factors and religiosity. Social and cultural expectations as well as access and availability may be the leading factors in behavioural change concerning traditional contraceptive use [16]. Differences in contraceptive use across Europe can also attribute to differences in gender inequality [24]. Particularly, country levels of gender equality are linked to the East-West divide in the type of contraceptive method used. Moreover, family policies may also play a role in decision-making about the method of contraceptive use. Facilitating the reconciliation of paid work and family life seems to enhance reproductive health [39, 40]. More attention for family policies may encourage modern contraceptive use [16]. This is particularly relevant for Eastern European countries like Romania and Bulgaria where development of family policies lags behind other Eastern European countries like Slovenia or the Czech Republic [41].

5. Conclusion

The main results could be summed up as follows: (1) The East-West divide in abortion behaviour was distorted, but not fully eliminated. Besides the former Eastern and Western abortion patterns, the new 'low abortion' pattern has emerged. (2) Within the EU countries, convergent trends towards lower abortion level were identified since 1990. However, as regards the structure of abortions, a pattern of divergence has been apparent due to differences in the transition to modern contraception use. (3) The use of modern methods of contraception rather depends on structural macro-level factors and contextual incentives and barriers as the impact of individual characteristics on the use of contraception does not differ much between countries under study.

Acknowledgements

The study was supported by the Czech Science Foundation project No.15-09443S.

Author details

Jiřina Kocourková
Department of Demography and Geodemography, Faculty of Science, Charles University, Prague, Czech Republic

*Address all correspondence to: jirina.kocourkova@natur.cuni.cz

References

[1] Blayo C. Les modes de prevention des naissances en Europe de l'Est. Population. 1991;**46**(3):527-546

[2] Troitskaia I, Avdeev A, Badurashvili I, Kapanadze E, Tretjakova V. Etude comparative des pratiques contraceptives: France, Górgie, Lithuanie et Russie. Revue d'études comparatives East-Ouest. 2009;**40**(3-4):241-272

[3] Agadjanian V. Is "abortion culture" fading in the former Soviet Union? Views about abortion and contraception in Kazakhstan. Studies in Family Planning. 2002;**33**:237-248

[4] Stloukal L. Understanding the "abortion culture" in Central and Eastern Europe. In: David HP, editor. From abortion to Contraception: A Resource to Public Policies and Reproductive Behaviour in Central and Eastern Europe from 1917 to the Present. Westport Connecticut: Greenwood Press; 1999. pp. 23-37

[5] Stloukal L. Demographic aspects of abortion in Eastern Europe: A study with special reference to the Czech Republic and Slovakia [doctor thesis]. The Australian National University; 1995. 420 p

[6] David HP, Popov AA. Russian Federation and USSR Successor States. In: David HP, editor. From Abortion to Contraception: A Resource to Public Policies and Reproductive Behaviour in Central and Eastern Europe from 1917 to the Present. Westport Connecticut: Greenwood Press; 1999. pp. 23-37

[7] Denisov BP, Sakevich VI, Jasilioniene A. Divergent trends in abortion and birth control practices in Belarus, Russia and Ukraine. PLoS One. 2012;7:1-10

[8] Frejka T. Birth regulation in Europe: Completing the contraceptive revolution. Demographic Research. 2008;**19**:73-84

[9] Westoff CF. Recent trends in abortion and contraception in 12 countries, DHS Analytical Studies no. 8. Calverton, Maryland, USA: ORC Macro; 2005. 64 p

[10] Westoff CF, Ryder NB. The Contraceptive Revolution. Princenton: Princenton: University Press; 1977

[11] Van de Kaa. Option and sequences: Europe's demographic patterns. Journal of the Australian Population Association. 1997;**14**(1):1-29

[12] Sobotka T. Re-emerging diversity: Rapid fertility change in Central and Eastern Europe after the collapse of the communist regimes. Population (English Edition). 2003;**58**(4-5):451-486

[13] Kocourková J, Fait T. Changes in contraceptive practice and the transition of reproduction pattern in the Czech population. The European Journal of Contraception and Reproductive Health Care. 2011;**16**(3):161-172

[14] Sedgh G, Bearak J, Singh S, et al. Abortion incidence between 1990 and 2014: Global, regional, and subregional levels and trends. The Lancet. 2016;**388**(1004):13-22

[15] Kocourková J. Relationship between abortion and contraception: A comparative socio-demographic analysis of Czech and Slovak populations. Women & Health. 2016;**56**(8):885-905

[16] Dereuddre R, Van de Putte B, Bracke P. Ready, willing, and able: Contraceptive use patterns across Europe. European Journal of Population. 2016a;**32**:543-573

[17] Sedgh G, Singh S, Henshaw KH, et al. Legal abortion Worldwide

in 2008: Levels and recent trends. Perspectives on Sexual and Reproductive Health. 2011;**43**(3):188-198

[18] Sedgh G, Singh S, Shah IH, Ahman E, Henshaw SK, Bankole A. Induced abortion: Incidence and trends worldwide from 1995 to 2008. The Lancet. 2012;**379**:625-632

[19] Guillaume A, Rossier C. Abortion Around the World. An: Overview of Legislation, Measures, Trends, and Consequences. Population (english edition). Institut National d'Études Démographiques (INED). 2018;**0**(2):217-306

[20] Cibula D. Women's contraceptive practices and sexual behaviour in Europe. The European Journal of Contraception and Reproductive Health Care. 2008;**13**(4):362-375

[21] Johnson S, Pion C, Jennings V. Current methods and attitudes of women towards contraception in Europe and America. Reproductive Health. 2013;**10**:7

[22] Skouby SO. Contraceptive use and behaviour in the 21st century: A comprehensive study across five European countries. The European Journal of Contraception and Reproductive Health Care. 2004;**9**(2):54-68

[23] Spinelli A, Talamanca IF, Lauria L. Patterns of contraceptive use in European countries. American Journal of Public Health. 2000;**90**(9):1403-1408

[24] Dereuddre R, Van de Velde S, Bracke P. Gender inequality and the "East-West" divide in contraception: An analysis at the individual, the couple, and the country level. Social Science & Medicine. 2016b;**161**:1-12

[25] Bongaarts J, Westoff CF. The potential role of contraception in reducing abortion. Studies in Family Planning. 2000;**31**:193-202

[26] Marston C, Cleland J. Relationships between contraception and abortion: A review of the evidence. International Family Planning Perspectives. 2003;**29**:6-13

[27] Westoff CF, Hammerslough CR, Paul L. The potential impact of improvements in contraception on fertility and abortion in Western countries. European Journal of Population/Revue européenne de Démographie. 1987;**3**:7-32

[28] Serbanescu F, Goldberg H, Morris L. Reproductive health in the transition countries of Europe. In: Macura et al., editors. The New Demographic Regime. Population Challenges and Policy Responses. Geneva: United Nations; 2005

[29] The Reproductive Health Report. The state of sexual and reproductive health within the European Union. The European Journal of Contraception & Reproductive Health Care. 2011;**16**(Suppl.1):S1-S70

[30] World Contraceptive Use. United Nations. 2011. Available from: https://www.un.org/en/development/desa/population/publications/family/contraceptive-wallchart-2011.asp

[31] GGP Data Archive. 2018. Generation and Gender Survey (Second Wave). Available from: http://www.ggp-i.org

[32] Vikat A, Spéder Z, Beets G, Billari FC, Bühler C, Désesquelles A, et al. Generations and gender survey (GGS): Towards a better understanding of relationships and processes in the life course. Demographic Research. 2007;**17**(14):389-439

[33] Isabel S, José Luis D, Iñaki L, et al. Contraceptive practices of women requesting induced abortion in Spain:

A cross-sectional multicentre study. The European Journal of Contraception & Reproductive Health Care. 2012;**17**(3):205-211

[34] Spéder Z, Kamarás F. Hungary: Secular fertility decline with distinct period fluctuations. Demographic Research. 2008;**19**:599-664

[35] Muresan C, Haragus PT, Haragus M, Schröder C. Romania: Childbearing metamorphosis within a changing context. Demographic Research. 2008;**19**:855-906

[36] Muresan C. Impact of induced abortion on fertility in Romania. European Journal of Population/ Revue européenne de Démographie. 2008;**24**:425-446

[37] Serbanescu F, Goldberg H, Morris L. Reproductive health in transition countries in the european context. Paper presented at the European Population Forum, Population Challenges and Policy Responses. Geneva; 2004

[38] Troitskaia I, Avdeev A. Recent features and factors of contraceptive use in Europe: Evidence from the Generation and Gender Survey. In: European Population Conference; 1.9.2010-4.9.2010; Vienna; 2010

[39] Clark R. Three faces of women's power and their reproductive health: A cross-national study. International Review of Modern Sociology. 2006;**32**(1):35-52

[40] Wang G. Reproductive health in the context of economic and democratic development. Comparative Sociology. 2004;**3**(2):135-162

[41] Frejka T, Basten S. Fertility and family policies in Central and Eastern Europe after 1990. Comparative Population Studies. 2016;**41**(1):3-56

Section 2

Practical Approaches to the Prediction, Prevention, and Treatment of Spontaneous Abortions

Chapter 4

Implantation and the Fetal Health

Aleksandar Ljubic, Dzihan Abazovic, Dusica Ljubic, Andrea Pirkovic and Andjela Perovic

Abstract

Implantation is one of the crucial periods in human reproduction. Increasing body of evidence suggests that the improper (dysfunctional) implantation and the formation of the placenta can endanger life and health of both the fetus and the mother, during prenatal life and decades after delivery. The idea of the inverted pyramid of prenatal care has emerged in the recent years, as the early detection and prevention of health disorders of the fetus are specially focusing on the first trimester. By applying this principle, disorders in the perinatal period could be prevented or treated with better outcome. The changes that lead to the deficient implantation should be sought in the preimplantation period, in relation between the embryo and the endometrium. It is possible that the time is approaching when the disorders of the pregnancy caused by dysfunctional implantation would be the indication for the application of a natural IVF (without ovarian stimulation) with the use of new biotechnological achievements. For better results of the perinatal medicine, it is necessary to apply earlier (in the preconception and preimplantation periods) the therapy based on the subcellular and genetic level by applying the latest biotechnological procedures.

Keywords: implantation, fetal health, pregnancy complications

1. Introduction

Most of the fetal and maternal complications become apparent with advancing gestation. However, since very important complications that occur later in pregnancy can be predicted in the first trimester, the focus has been set on the evaluations in early pregnancy, thus inverting the pyramid of prenatal care. Although vast majority of early screening tests have been developed and employed, the outcome of pregnancies with the major obstetric syndromes still fails to be significantly improved. The changes etiologically and pathophysiologically associated with disturbed placentation and responsible for the perinatal mortality and morbidity should be sought even earlier, in the preimplantation period, in relation between the embryo and the endometrium.

2. Early pregnancy screening tests and algorithms

The idea of inverted pyramid of prenatal care has emerged for the purpose of prediction and prevention and then early detection and treatment of health disorders of the fetus. By applying this principle, a number of disorders could be prevented or treated with better outcome: fetal aneuploidy and anomalies, miscarriage, stillbirth, preterm delivery, preterm premature rupture of membranes, preeclampsia, and intrauterine growth restriction [1].

In recent years, screening for aneuploidies during the first trimester has reached effectiveness of over 90% in identifying the most common aneuploidies by a combination of maternal age, fetal nuchal translucency, as well as analysis of free beta-hCG and pregnancy-associated plasma protein A (PAPP-A) [2]. Effectiveness of screening for potential aneuploidies was further augmented with the introduction of the noninvasive prenatal testing using maternal plasma cell-free (cf) DNA, as a secondary test in those patients already regarded as being at high risk. The detection rate of major aneuploidies with this test is up to 99. 3%, with false positive rate of 0. 11% [3].

The development of sonography and MRI diagnostics has led to a growing number of early detected anomalies. A large number of these anomalies can be detected already at 11–14 weeks, while a number can only be found at a later gestation [4]. The prenatal detection rate for the major anomalies is around 68% (varying from 33 to 96%) [5, 6].

First trimester screening often focuses on fetal aneuploidy and major structural anomalies. However, certain maternal characteristics, such as the age and body mass index (BMI), have shown to be very informative, with regard to the predicting miscarriage and stillbirth. The risk of preterm delivery is determined by algorithms that combine these results of the first trimester screening for aneuploidy, increased nuchal translucency, the abnormal ductus venosus flow, and low level of PAPP-A, with the characteristics of the mother [7–9]. Such example is the information on the length of the cervical canal from 11- to 13-week gestation [9, 10]. The risk of spontaneous preterm delivery is associated with cervical shortening in the second trimester, as well as in the first trimester. Combining this parameter with fetal aneuploidy analyses and major structural anomaly results is likely to be used in the future to select a high-risk group that may benefit from close follow-up.

Another example is the screening for the development of early preeclampsia (PE), based on the combination of maternal risk factors, mean arterial pressure, maternal serum PAPP-A, uterine artery Doppler, and placental growth factor. This algorithm has a 95% detection rate for a false-positive rate of 10% [11, 12]. Also, different angiogenesis-related biomarkers; antiangiogenic proteins, like soluble fms-like tyrosine kinase-1 (sFlt-1) and soluble endoglin; or proangiogenic proteins, placenta growth factor (PlGF) and vascular endothelial growth factor (VEGF) have been pointed out by a number of authors [10]. The placental protein-13 and other markers, disintegrin and metalloprotease-12 (ADAM12), activin A, or inhibin A, and other microelements or antioxidants, in isolation or in combination, were evaluated in order to predict complications of pregnancy [13–15]. It was also shown that early administration of low-dose aspirin (60–80 mg), starting from the first trimester, reduces the incidence of intrauterine growth restriction as well as its related pregnancy and neonatal complications for 17%, with number needed to treat (NNT) 72, and 14% reduction in fetal or neonatal deaths with NNT 24 [16].

The detection of the small for gestational age (SGA) fetuses could be predicted by algorithms with the combination of maternal characteristics, mean arterial pressure, uterine artery Doppler, and the measurement of various placental products in maternal blood at 11–13 weeks, at a false-positive rate of 10%, about 75% of pregnancies without preeclampsia delivering SGA neonates before 37 weeks and 45% of those delivering at term [17]. Screening for macrosomia by a combination of maternal characteristics and obstetric history with fetal NT and maternal serum-free ß-hCG and PAPP-A at 11–13 weeks could potentially identify, at a false-positive rate of 10%, about 35% of women who deliver macrosomic neonates [18].

Despite the introduction of the vast early pregnancy screening tests, there is still a very slight decrease or even increase in the rate of preterm birth and almost a constant rate of miscarriage, stillbirth, preeclampsia, and SGA [19–23]. Except for hereditary and structural disorders of the fetus, other disorders are etiologically and pathophysiologically associated with disturbed placentation and responsible for the perinatal mortality and morbidity [24].

The reasons why the modern medicine still fails to significantly improve the outcome of pregnancy with the major obstetric syndromes should be sought in the earlier period of pregnancy, even before the conception, and on another subcellular level (Personal communication Dudenhausen, Tirana 2015). Because the consequence of these disturbances is seen in dysfunctional placentation, their sources must be searched before the time of implantation. This means that the changes that lead to the insufficient implantation should be sought in the preimplantation period, in relation between the embryo and the endometrium.

The onset and progression of pregnancy require the coordinated implantation of the embryo and trophoblast invasion into the receptive maternal decidua, followed by proper remodeling of the spiral arteries. Proliferation, migration, and invasion of trophoblastic cells into the maternal endometrium are the essential steps. If any of these steps fails to complete properly because of the endometrial dysfunction, the consequences would be the basis for development of obstetric complications.

3. Maternal health at preconception period

The implanting embryo physically establishes connections with the mother through the endometrium, by a fine-tuned and synchronized crosstalk necessary to support the feto-placental development and health throughout gestation [25]. Early alterations of endometrial physiology can affect the development of the conceptus and the success of pregnancy. The overall status of maternal health is reflecting on the endometrium. If we agree that the optimally prepared mucous membranes (either endogenously, by its own sex hormone or by exogenous regimes) are one of the preconditions for the successful implantation, then the modification of its preparation could influence the occurrence of disorders in later pregnancy and after the birth of the child.

Several studies have shown that preimplantation embryos are sensitive to environmental conditions in which it develops, either in vitro or in vivo, for example, in response to culture conditions or maternal diet [26]. Those conditions can affect future growth and developmental potential, both pre- and postnatally. Recent findings have demonstrated that perturbations of the maternal physiology during the peri-conceptional period (e.g., maternal diet) have impact both on preimplantation phenotype and long-term development and could lead to impaired health during adulthood [26]. Emerging evidence suggests the metabolic status of the mother may "program" the offspring's long-term risk of metabolic disease [27].

Modifications of preimplantation embryo conditions, using assisted reproductive technologies (ARTs) or somatic cell nuclear transfer (SCNT), have been associated with developmental abnormalities and postnatal consequences such as the large offspring syndrome (LOS) in animals [28–30]. Early alterations of the maternal or embryo environment may affect the quality of the embryo-endometrium crosstalk that further leads to pregnancy failure or postnatal detrimental consequences.

4. Endometrium

Before the embryo can implant in the endometrium, the endometrium must be in a receptive state. As a result of a series of timed hormonal events, the so-called window of implantation is opened, which is the time most suitable for the endometrium to support trophoblast-endometrial interaction [31].

The term windows of vulnerability (WOV), i.e., period of time when the endometrium is subject to the influence of factors that may disrupt implantation conditions, has recently been introduced within the framework of reproductive medicine, besides the window of implantation (WOI), i.e., the optimal period of time of activation of endometrial receptivity (De Ziegler, personal communication, MSD symposium, Barcelona 2016).

Prepregnancy approaches such as weight management, blood pressure and blood sugar control, smoking cessation, and optimization of the pregnancy interval may improve implantation and placentation and lead to better pregnancy outcomes [32].

There are a number of different treatment protocols for the "inadequate" endometrium. The medical treatment with estrogens, vasodilators, and sildenafil citrate has neither led to significant improvements of morphological parameters nor to the results in terms of increasing implantation and reduction of the number of miscarriages [33, 34]. There have been reports of trials with immunoglobulins and anticoagulants in pregnancy complication prevention [35–39].

The local endometrium therapy is ongoing for several years. One of the promising therapeutic targets is the corticotropin-releasing hormone (CRH). During implantation, corticotropin-releasing hormone plays a key role in facilitating endometrial decidualization and early maternal tolerance. The embryo implantation provokes the maternal endometrial response similar to the invading semi-allograft that produces acute inflammatory response. After the implantation, the embryo suppresses this response and prevents the rejection [40]. The deregulation of expression pattern of CRH was associated with unfavorable reproductive outcomes as well as chronic endometrium-derived inflammatory disorders, such as endometriosis and adenomyosis [41]. Positive outcome was found after the intrauterine administration of autologous peripheral blood mononuclear cells (PBMCs) [41] especially when pretreated with corticotropin-releasing hormone that acts by regulating apoptosis of activated T- lymphocytes at the implantation site [42]. The results of eight studies showed that intrauterine administration of activated autologous peripheral blood mononuclear cells prior to embryo transfer improves the reproductive outcomes in women with repeated implantation failure [43].

Besides endometrial receptivity, another very important parameter is the endometrial thickness. Defined minimal thickness at approximately 7 mm and clinical pregnancy rates after embryo transfer increase with increasing endometrial thickness. One of the new therapeutic approaches to improve endometrial thickness is the intrauterine perfusion with granulocyte colony-stimulating factor (G-CSF). In clinical reproduction, G-CSF has been proposed as a treatment for implantation failure and repeated miscarriages, two indications for which a US patent has been issued. These authors have applied the drug subcutaneously [44]. Gleicher's papers on flushing uterus cavity with growth factors before the embryo transfer have proposed granulocyte colony-stimulating factor as the treatment of implantation failure and repeated miscarriages [44]. Chang reported successful endometrial expansion in a small group of women with thin endometrium resistant to standard treatments, who were able to proceed to embryo transfer and conceive after uterine perfusion with G-CSF [45].

The use of platelet-rich plasma (PRP) to improve endometrial receptivity is gaining increasing attention in assisted reproduction technologies. Platelets contain a significant amount of growth factors that have positive effects on local tissue repair and endometrial receptivity. Several authors have reported autologous PRP intrauterine injection improves pregnancy and birth rates, especially in patients presenting poor endometrial growth [46].

Chang and associates have recently published the attempt to improve the quality of endometrial thickness, implantation rate, and pregnancy success and to reduce the complications and miscarriage rate, by flushing the uterus cavity with autologous platelet-rich plasma in preparation for the implantation during IVF process [47]. Farimani reported the first successful pregnancy after administration of PRP in a woman with recurrent implantation failure [48]. Kim et al. suggested that the use of autologous PRP improved not only endometrial thickness but restored the endometrial receptivity of damaged endometrium and increased the implantation, pregnancy, and live birth rates (LBR) of the 24 patients with refractory thin endometrium [49]. This therapy delivers biological growth factors, PDGF, TGF-b, and VEGF, insulin-like growth factor 1, epidermal growth factor (EGF), and epithelial cell growth factor to the endometrium. Our group has, so far, treated 25 patients with PRP technology and has achieved a significant improvement of the implantation rates and in reducing the number of abortions. We reported the first case of human embryo obtained after autologous platelet leukocyte-rich plasma (PLRP) in vitro activation of ovaries by interrupting Hippo signaling and PLRP stimulating AKT pathway with ultrasound-guided orthotropic re-transplantation [50]. The patient was a case of an early menopausal woman for whom the ovarian cortex was frozen, thawed, and treated with autologous PLRP which was then transplanted into her menopausal ovaries. Two months after the procedure, follicle formation was noted, and an egg was retrieved resulting in a single embryo [50].

The human endometrium is a dynamic tissue that undergoes monthly cyclic changes, including proliferation, differentiation, and degeneration. Apoptosis is the common pathway of cell death for eliminating senescent endometrial cells from the functional layer of the human endometrium during the late secretory phases of the cycle. It has recently been implied that autophagy is involved in the endometrial cell cycle affecting apoptosis and is the most prominent during the late secretory phase [51]. It is known that the impact on autophagy processes in the endometrium may lead to a reduced incidence of pregnancy complications related to the implantation. Our group has proved that autophagy, a process of controlled self-digestion involved in cellular homeostasis, is dysregulated in endometrial tissue of polycystic ovary syndrome (PCOS) patients and that treatment with metformin might influence endometrial autophagy in PCOS [52]. Other studies reported that metformin can improve endometrial receptivity, enhance endometrial vascularity and blood flow, and revert endometrial hyperplasia and carcinoma into normal endometria in addition to improving hyperandrogenism and insulin resistance in some women with PCOS [53, 54].

5. Embryo environment

The essential requirements for normal implantation and subsequent placentation leading to a healthy gestation are receptive endometrium and healthy embryo. However, there is still a growing number of unexplained failed implantation outcomes that could not be assigned to known factors and require further investigation.

In recent years it was indicated that different etiologies of infertility arose as a result of the underlying genetic and epigenetic changes that contribute to the endometrial dysfunction and lead to implantation failure, miscarriage, and adverse outcomes. These epigenetic and genetic changes lead to placentation defects and contribute to the short- and long-term outcomes associated with infertility. One of the main causes for altered genetic and epigenetic regulation of embryo development and placentation was assigned to hormonal and nutrition-related changes in maternal environment. Embryos respond to the in vivo maternal environment during gestation or during cultivation in vitro in multiple ways that can influence their future growth and health. Developmental plasticity could be altered by the changes in imprinted gene expression, nutrient, and stress-related signaling pathways or cell cycling and apoptotic rates. Embryo phenotype changes through a complex network of interactions with a central role for maternal-fetal neuroendocrine signaling [55]. Maternal undernutrition during gestation alters maternal steroid hormone levels, including elevation of glucocorticoids (GC; corticosterone, cortisol), the stress hormones, which can alter the physiological condition of the conceptus and affect the intrauterine fetal and postnatal growth and cardiovascular and metabolic physiology and enhance the risk of adult-onset disease. This exposure of the embryo to glucocorticoids can alter the fetal hypothalamus pituitary adrenal (HPA) axis, leading to increased fetal GC activity which can, in turn, modify the expression of many downstream-regulated genes that control growth and metabolism, including cardiovascular and renal physiology [55].

The influence of placental function and placental/fetal exchange on fetal programming has been in focus of the recent research. Now it has become widely accepted that maternal nutrition can have the long-term consequences on the offspring without necessarily affecting the size at birth. Altered embryo phenotypes induced by prenatal nutrition are associated with epigenetic modifications. Many imprinted genes contribute to placental function and nutrient exchange [56]. Early epigenetic effects in embryos caused by environmental conditions can lead to physiological impairment to growth due to reduced nutrient supply. There is now evidence from human studies and animal experiments that show the overnutrition and undernutrition during the prenatal period which have lifelong health effects for the offspring and induce the development of noncommunicable diseases during postnatal life [57].

Besides nutrition, the hormonal milieu at conception is known to affect a number of imprinted genes that are expressed during the preimplantation period. Hormonal status will be especially affected during fertility treatment, mostly during IVF. Because superovulation could lead to altered expression of endometrial genes critical to tissue remodeling and placentation, hyperstimulated hormonal status has been implicated in an increased risk for pregnancy complications related to abnormal placentation [58]. Although global methylation pattern was found to be similar among the IVF and spontaneous conceptions early during placentation in the first trimester, differential methylation has been identified in multiple loci between IVF and non-IVF fertility treatments pregnancies but not when compared with spontaneous conceptions. This suggests that there are differences in the infertile population that might be linked to specific treatments, including the hormonal hyperstimulation, that could affect gene imprinting [59]. Several studies have found that the use of ARTs is linked with irregular DNA methylation in human gamete, embryo, placenta, and umbilical cord samples [60, 61]. There were also studies that showed association between specific procedures with methylation differences in placenta, suggesting that specific fertility treatments affect the placental epigenome and function [62].

6. Embryo monitoring

The embryo has, in addition to the endometrium, the crucial importance for the success and regularity of the implantation and then placentation. The morphological assessment of the embryos' quality is insufficient for the cognition of its biological resources. The new invasive and noninvasive techniques of embryo quality assessment have been developed. Nowadays, the invasive technology means preimplantation genetic testing (PGT), the aneuploidy screening, or diagnosis of specific genetic disorders of the embryo before the transfer by using next-generation sequencing (NGS). These tests include biopsy trophectoderm cells with blastocyst vitrification [63–65]. With trophectoderm biopsy, both maternal and paternal abnormalities can be studied. Possible disadvantages are the presence of mosaicism and the fact that the trophectoderm might not be a representative of the inner cell mass.

Noninvasive time-lapse embryo monitoring allows continuous embryo observation without the need to remove the embryo from optimal culturing conditions. The information on the cleavage pattern, morphologic changes, and embryo development dynamics could help us identify embryos with a higher implantation potential. It has also been shown that imaging phenotypes reflect the molecular program of the embryo, where individual blastomeres develop autonomously toward embryo genomic activation [66].

This type of monitoring allows for the collection of much more information on the timing of the cleavages and the dynamics of the morphologic changes, with analysis of the kinetics of the events up until the blastocyst stage [67].

Various kinetic and morphologic markers have already been found that are associated with the minimal likelihood of implantation and others that are predictive of blastocyst development, implantation potential, genetic health, and pregnancy [68, 69].

7. Gametes

After the formation of the embryo, its fate is already determined. The gamete quality has the crucial part in the creation of the high-quality embryos. The conditions, in which oogenesis and spermatogenesis take place, have a crucial impact on the quality of embryos that is formed from these gametes.

7.1 Oogenesis

The evaluation of the oocyte quality based on morphological evaluation is not sufficient for an insight into the biological potential. It can identify those cells that have nuclear immaturity, significant degeneration, or major abnormalities. Recently, the developed strategies including the genomic, transcriptomic, and proteomic approaches have been applied in assisted reproduction. Their goal is to identify a "molecular profile" of embryo development by detecting the chemical components in the oocyte, granulosa cells, follicular fluid, and embryo culture medium [70].

Better predictors, the birefringence properties of the meiotic spindle, and the zona pellucida are indicative of good health of the oocyte [71]. A very useful data can be obtained from the application of studying gene expression from cumulus cells, using microarrays, as biomarkers for oocyte viability. The metabolomic profiling of oocyte spent culture media by mass spectroscopy has shown differences related to oocyte maturation, embryo development, and implantation success [72]. Oocyte quality can be assessed by the measurement of oocyte oxygen consumption [73].

Spermatogenesis: the quality of spermatogenesis is the condition for the formation of a good embryo. The advanced sperm selection techniques are based not only on the morphological assessment (defragmentation, MACS) but also on the evaluation of specific cellular characteristics (membrane integrity, density, surface charge) that provide a choice of better quality sperm. The methods of improving conditions of gametogenesis, which are applied so far, do not provide a sufficient effect. They are mainly related to the balance correction of microelements and vitamins, as well as the oxydo-reductive processes in the body. The sperm chromatin and DNA integrity are necessary to ensure normal embryo development. It is now clear that DNA damage in spermatozoa has a negative influence on blastocyst development and the pregnancy outcome [74] . Similarly, centrosome integrity is critical for successful fertilization and embryo development. There are studies that have described the association between sperm with DNA damage and a history of recurrent miscarriage [75].

7.2 Advanced therapy

Magnetic-activated cell sorting (MACS) technology for sperm could improve obstetric and perinatal outcomes compared with those achieved after swim up. Treatment of sperm with MACS procedure prior to IVF results in a marked improvement in pregnancy rate and cessation of the abortion rate in couples whose ejaculates initially had high levels of SDF [76].

A number of prerequisites are needed to create high-quality oocytes, those conditions are likely to be grouped into several parts: the existence of high quality responsive oogonia, its potential of the adequate number increase and quality of mitochondria, the presence of sufficient amounts and types of growth factors, orchestrated by the balance of blocking (Hippo) and activating (ACT) gene pathways [77].

For decades it was believed that the woman's reproductive potential is entirely dependent on the size of the stock (pool) of primordial follicles in the ovary. The paradigm that has prevailed for decades in the scientific world about the existence of a consistent number of primordial follicles, established during embryonic and fetal period, was in many ways changed by Tilly's group work. They practically demonstrated the existence of germline or oogonial stem cells [78].

Their dormant status is characterized by communication with surrounding granulosa cells and numerous mechanical and chemical factors controlling the progression of their cell cycle. These factors control signaling activation of the pathways included in the primordial follicle dormant status regulation, like Hippo and AKT signaling [77]. During the recent years, various programs have been developed to try to improve the quality of oocytes. It has been shown that it can be influenced on the activation of primordial cells and maturation to the mature oocyte. The stem cells can be influenced by the stem cell therapy in order to obtain the intracellular communication with the existing ovarian primordial oogonia. The therapy with mesenchymal stem cells has led to the recovery features of oocytes after the chemotherapy-induced insufficiency [79]. The animal experiments by the in vitro therapy with developed stem cells have led to the birth of live offspring without abnormalities [80]. Other groups of authors have tried to improve the ovarian function with the growth factors obtained from the plasma and enriched with platelets and leukocytes. The cases of childbirth after re-transplantation of ovaries with support of PRP have been published [81]. Our group has achieved a normal pregnancy outcome after the sonographically guided therapy with growth factors in a female patient aged 40 years, after 18 attempts of in vitro fertilization.

The role of the number and function of mitochondria in the development of quality oocytes is surely very important. The problems of mitochondrial heteroplasmy go with the complicated, technologically very complex methods of polar body transfer, spindle transfer, and pronuclear or oocyte transfer [82–84]. The augmentation of autologous mitochondria carries a potential treatment. Our team has inaugurated the attempt of the mitochondrial energy boosting with ovarian high-intensity interval training (HIIT).

The autologous growth factors that are intraovarian instilled are leading to the changes in the production and efficiency of the local growth factors. The influence on the genetic control of oogenesis, by the modification of the Hippo and AKT signaling pathways, is possible in different ways. The correction of the gene signaling or autologous tissue genetic bioengineering is certainly a step forward in obtaining the quality gametes [50, 84].

8. Conclusion

Implantation is one of the crucial periods in human reproduction. Increasing body of evidence suggests that the improper (dysfunctional) implantation and the formation of the placenta can endanger life and health of both the fetus and the mother, during prenatal life and decades after delivery. The changes that lead to the insufficient implantation should be sought in the preimplantation period, in relation between the embryo and the endometrium. It is possible that the time is approaching when the disorders of the pregnancy caused by dysfunctional implantation would be the indication for the application of a natural IVF (without ovarian stimulation) with the use of new biotechnological achievements. For better results of the perinatal medicine, it is necessary to apply earlier (in the preconception and preimplantation periods) the therapy based on the subcellular and genetic level by applying the latest biotechnological procedures.

Author details

Aleksandar Ljubic[1], Dzihan Abazovic[2], Dusica Ljubic[3], Andrea Pirkovic[4*] and Andjela Perovic[4]

1 Medigroup, Belgrade, Serbia

2 Renova Clinic, Belgrade, Serbia

3 Special Gynecology Hospital Jevremova, Belgrade, Serbia

4 Segova Biotechnology, Belgrade, Serbia

*Address all correspondence to: andreapirkovic@segova.com

References

[1] Nicolaides K. A model for a new pyramid of prenatal care based on the 11 to 13 weeks' assessment. Prenatal Diagnosis. 2011;**31**:3-6

[2] Wright D, Syngelaki A, Bradbury I, Akolekar R, Nicolaides KH. First-trimester screening for trisomies 21, 18 and 13 by ultrasound and biochemical testing. Fetal Diagnosis and Therapy. 2014;**35**(2):118-126. DOI: 10.1159/000357430. Epub 2013 Dec 18

[3] Sonek JD, Cuckle HS. What will be the role of first-trimester ultrasound if cell-free DNA screening for aneuploidy becomes routine? Ultrasound in Obstetrics & Gynecology. 2014;**44**:621-630

[4] Renna MD, Pisani P, Conversano F, et al. Sonographic markers for early diagnosis of fetal malformations. World Journal of Radiology. 2013;**5**(10):356-371

[5] Stoll C, Clementi M, Euroscan Study Group. Prenatal diagnosis of dysmorphic syndromes by routine fetal ultrasound examination across Europe. Ultrasound in Obstetrics & Gynecology. 2003;**21**(6):543-551

[6] Rydberg C, Tunón K. Detection of fetal abnormalities by second-trimester ultrasound screening in a non-selected population. Acta Obstetricia et Gynecologica Scandinavica. 2017;**96**(2):176-182. DOI: 10.1111/aogs.13037. Epub 2016 Nov 22

[7] Datta MR, Raut A. Efficacy of first-trimester ultrasound parameters for prediction of early spontaneous abortion. International Journal of Gynaecology and Obstetrics. 2017;**138**(3):325-330

[8] Wu Y, He J, Guo C, et al. Serum biomarker analysis in patients with recurrent spontaneous abortion. Molecular Medicine Reports. 2017;**16**(3):2367-2378

[9] Greco E, Lange A, Ushakov F, Rodriguez Calvo J, Nicolaides KH. Prediction of spontaneous preterm delivery from endocervical length at 11 to 13 weeks. Prenatal Diagnosis. 2011;**31**(1):84-89

[10] Conde-Agudelo A, Romero R. Predictive accuracy of changes in transvaginal sonographic cervical length over time for preterm birth: A systematic review and metaanalysis. American Journal of Obstetrics and Gynecology. 2015;**213**(6):789-780

[11] Poon NC, Nicolaides K. Early prediction of preeclampsia. Obstetrics and Gynecology International. 2014;**1**:1-11

[12] Akolekar R, Syngelaki A, Sarquis R, Zvanca M, Nicolaides KH. Prediction of early, intermediate and late pre-eclampsia from maternal factors, biophysical and biochemical markers at 11-13 weeks. Prenatal Diagnosis. 2011b;**31**(1):66-74

[13] Mihailović M, Cvetković M, Ljubić A, et al. Selenium and malondialdehyde content and glutathione peroxidase activity in maternal and umbilical cord blood and amniotic fluid. Biological Trace Element Research. 2000;**73**(1):47-54

[14] Ćetković A, Ljubić A, Patterson M, et al. Plasma kisspeptin levels in pregnancies with diabetes and hypertensive disease as a potential marker of placental dysfunction and adverse perinatal outcome. Endocrine Research. 2012;**37**(2):78-88

[15] Giguère Y, Charland M, et al. Combining biochemical and

ultrasonographic markers in predicting preeclampsia: A systematic review. Clinical Chemistry. 2010;**56**(3):361-375

[16] Duley L, Henderson-Smart DJ, Meher S, King JF. Antiplatelet agents in preventing pre-eclampsia. Cohrane. 2007;**2**. Article No: CD004659. DOI: 10.1002/14651858.CD004659.pub2.

[17] Karagiannis G, Akolekar R, Sarquis R, Wright D, Nicolaides K. Prediction of small-for-gestation neonates from biophysical and biochemical markers at 11-13 weeks. Fetal Diagnosis and Therapy. 2011;**29**(2):148-154

[18] Poon LC1, Karagiannis G, Stratieva V, Syngelaki A, Nicolaides KH. First-trimester prediction of macrosomia. Fetal Diagnosis and Therapy. 2011;**29**(2):139-147

[19] Baltaci V, Baltaci E. Genetic aspects of recurrent miscarriages. JSM Invitro Fertilization. 2016;**1**(1):1002

[20] Chabra S. Estimates of perinatal death: A global initiative! Journal of Perinatology. 2017;**37**:1248

[21] Rolnik DL, O'Gorman N, Roberge, et al. Early screening and prevention of preterm pre-eclampsia with aspirin: Time for clinical implementation. Ultrasound in Obstetrics & Gynecology. 2017;**50**:551-556

[22] Gregory ECW, MacDorman MF, Martin JA. Trends in Fetal and Perinatal Mortality in the United States, 2006-2012. NCHS Data Brief, No 169. Hyattsville, MD: National Center for Health Statistics; 2014

[23] Ananth V, Keyes K, Wapner RJ. Pre-eclampsia rates in the United States, 1980-2010: Age-period-cohort analysis. British Medical Journal. 2013;**347**:6564

[24] Ljubić A. Inverted pyramid of prenatal care—is it enough? Should it be—extended inverted pyramid of prenatal care?. Journal of Perinatal Medicine. 2017;**46**(7):716-720

[25] Mansouri-Attia N, Sandra O, Aubert J, Degrelle S, Everts RE, Giraud-Delville C, et al. Endometrium as an early sensor of in vitro embryo manipulation technologies. Proceedings of the National Academy of Sciences of the United States of America. 2009;**106**(14):5687-5692. DOI: 10.1073/pnas.0812722106

[26] Fleming TP et al. The embryo and its future. Biology of Reproduction. 2004;**71**:1046-1054

[27] Price S, Nankervis A, Permezel M, Prendergast L, Sumithran P, Proietto J. Health consequences for mother and baby of substantial pre-conception weight loss in obese women: Study protocol for a randomized controlled trial. Trials. 2018;**19**(1):248. DOI: 10.1186/s13063-018-2615-6

[28] Sinclair KD. Assisted reproductive technologies and pregnancy outcomes: Mechanistic insights from animal studies. Seminars in Reproductive Medicine. 2008;**26**:153-161

[29] Constant F et al. Large offspring or large placenta syndrome? Morphometric analysis of late gestation bovine placentomes from somatic nuclear transfer pregnancies complicated by hydroallantois. Biology of Reproduction. 2006;**75**:122-130

[30] Lazzari G et al. Cellular and molecular deviations in bovine in vitro-produced embryos are related to the large offspring syndrome. Biology of Reproduction. 2002;**67**:767-775

[31] Casper RF, Yanushpolsky EH. Optimal endometrial preparation for frozen embryo transfer cycles: Window of implantation and progesterone support. Fertility and Sterility. 2016;**105**(4):867-872

[32] Urato AC, Norwitz ER. A guide towards pre-pregnancy management of defective implantation and placentation. Best Practice & Research: Clinical Obstetrics and Gynaecology. 2011;**25**:367-387

[33] Shen MS, Wang CW, Chen CH, Tzeng CR. New horizon on successful management for a woman with repeated implantation failure due to unresponsive thin endometrium: Use of extended estrogen supplementation. Journal of Obstetrics and Gynaecology Research. 2013;**39**(5):1092-1094

[34] Stephenson MD, Fluker MR. Treatment of repeated unexplained in vitro fertilization failure with intravenous immunoglobulin: A randomized, placebo-controlled Canadian trial. Fertility and Sterility. 2000;**74**:1108-1113

[35] Stern C, Chamley L, Norris H, Hale L, Baker HW. A randomized, double-blind, placebo-controlled trial of heparin and aspirin for women with in vitro fertilization implantation failure and antiphospholipid or antinuclear antibodies. Fertility and Sterility. 2003;**80**:376-383

[36] Boomsma CM, Keay SD, Macklon NS. Peri-implantation glucocorticoid administration for assisted reproductive technology cycles. Cochrane The Cochrane Database of Systematic Reviews. 2007 Article No: CD005996. DOI: 10.1002/14651858. CD005996.pub3

[37] Gelbaya TA, Kyrgiou M, Li TC, Stern C, Nardo LG. Low-dose aspirin for in vitro fertilization: A systematic review and meta-analysis. Human Reproduction Update. 2007;**13**:357-364

[38] Mekinian A, Cohen J, Alijotas-Reig J, et al. Unexplained recurrent miscarriage and recurrent implantation failure: Is there a place for immunomodulation? American Journal of Reproductive Immunology. 2016;**76**(1):8-28

[39] Yu N, Zhang B, Xu M, et al. Intrauterine administration of autologous peripheral blood mononuclear cells(PBMCs) activated by HCG improves the implantation and pregnancy rates in patients with repeated implantation failure: A prospective randomized study. American Journal of Reproductive Immunology. 2016;**76**(3):212-216

[40] Kalantaridou SN, Zoumakis E, Makrigiannakis A, Godoy H, Chrousos GP. The role of corticotropin-releasing hormone in blastocyst implantation and early fetal immunotolerance. Hormone and Metabolic Research. 2007;**39**(6):474-477

[41] Antonis M, Moncef B, Thomas V, Sami M, Sophia K, Timur G. Repeated implantation failure: A new potential treatment option. European Journal of Clinical Investigation. 2015;**45**:380-384. DOI: 10.1111/eci.12417

[42] Wurfel W. Treatment with granulocyte colony-stimulating factor in patients with repetitive implantation failures and/or recurrent spontaneous abortions. Journal of Reproductive Immunology. 2015;**108**:123-135

[43] Maleki-Hajiagha A, Razavi M, Rezaeinejad M, Rouholamin S, Almasi-Hashiani A, Pirjani R, et al. Intrauterine administration of autologous peripheral blood mononuclear cells in patients with recurrent implantation failure: A systematic review and meta-analysis. Journal of Reproductive Immunology. 2019;**131**:50-56

[44] Gleicher N, Vidali A, Barad DH. Successful treatment of unresponsive thin endometrium. Fertility and Sterility. 2011;**95**(6):2123

[45] Chang Y, Li J, Chen Y, et al. Autologous platelet-rich plasma promotes endometrial growth and

improves pregnancy outcome during in vitro fertilization. International Journal of Clinical and Experimental Medicine. 2015;**8**(1):1286-1290

[46] Bos-Mikich A, Ferreira MO, de Oliveira R, Frantz N. Platelet-rich plasma or blood-derived products to improve endometrial receptivity? Journal of Assisted Reproduction and Genetics. 2019;**36**(4):613-620. DOI: 10.1007/s10815-018-1386-z

[47] Sumarac-Dumanovic M, Apostolovic M, Janjetovic K, et al. Downregulation of autophagy gene expression in endometria from women with polycystic ovary syndrome. Molecular and Cellular Endocrinology. 2016;**440**:116-124

[48] Farimani M, Poorolajal J, Rabiee S, Bahmanzadeh M. Successful pregnancy and live birth after intrauterine administration of autologous platelet-rich plasma in a woman with recurrent implantation failure: A case report. International Journal of Reproductive BioMedicine (Yazd). 2017;**15**(12):803-806

[49] Kim H, Shin JE, Koo HS, Kwon H, Choi DH, Kim JH. Effect of autologous platelet-rich plasma treatment on refractory thin endometrium during the frozen embryo transfer cycle: A pilot study. Frontiers in Endocrinology (Lausanne). 2019;**10**:61. Published 2019 Feb 14. DOI: 10.3389/fendo.2019.00061

[50] Ljubić A, Abazović D, Vučetić D, et al. Autologous ovarian in vitro activation with ultrasound-guided orthotopic re-transplantation (in press). American Journal of Clinical and Experimental Obstetrics and Gynecology. 2017;**4**(5):51-57

[51] Choi JY, Jo MW, Lee EY, Oh YK, Choi DS. The role of autophagy in human endometrium. Biology of Reproduction. 2012;**86**(3):70. DOI: 10.1095/biolreprod.111.096206

[52] Schoolcraft WB, Fragouli E, Stevens J, Munne S, Katz-Jaffe MG, Wells D. Clinical application of comprehensive chromosomal screening at the blastocyst stage. Fertility and Sterility. 2010;**94**:1700-1706

[53] Jakubowicz DJ, Seppala M, Jakubowicz S, Rodriguez-Armas O, Rivas-Santiago A, Koistinen H, et al. Insulin reduction with metformin increases luteal phase serum glycodelin and insulin-like growth factor-binding protein 1 concentrations and enhances uterine vascularity and blood flow in the polycystic ovary syndrome. The Journal of Clinical Endocrinology and Metabolism. 2001;**86**:1126-1133

[54] Palomba S, Russo T, Orio F Jr, Falbo A, Manguso F, Cascella T, et al. Uterine effects of metformin administration in anovulatory women with polycystic ovary syndrome. Human Reproduction. 2006;**21**:457-465

[55] Bertram CE, Hanson MA. Prenatal programming of postnatal endocrine responses by glucocorticoids. Reproduction. 2002;**124**:459-467

[56] Lucifero D, Chaillet JR, Trasler JM. Potential significance of genomic imprinting defects for reproduction and assisted reproductive technology. Human Reproduction Update. 2004;**10**:3-18

[57] Velazquez MA, Sun C, Fleming TP. Chapter 6—Parental nutrition and developmental origins of health and disease. In: Rosenfeld CS, editor. The Epigenome and Developmental Origins of Health and Disease. Academic Press, Elsevier; 2016. pp. 89-102. ISBN 9780128013830. DOI: 10.1016/B978-0-12-801383-0.00006-2

[58] Senapati S, Wang F, Ord T, Coutifaris C, Feng R, Mainigi M. Superovulation alters the expression of endometrial genes critical to tissue

remodeling and placentation. Journal of Assisted Reproduction and Genetics. 2018;**35**(10):1799-1808

[59] Pisarska MD, Chan JL, Lawrenson K, Gonzalez TL, Wang ET. Genetics and epigenetics of infertility and treatments on outcomes. The Journal of Clinical Endocrinology & Metabolism. 2019;**104**(6):1871-1886. DOI: 10.1210/jc.2018-01869

[60] Hajj N, Haaf T. Epigenetic disturbances in in vitro cultured gametes and embryos: Implications for human assisted reproduction. Fertility and Sterility. 2013;**99**(3):632-641

[61] Nelissen EC, Dumoulin JC, Daunay A, Evers JL, Tost J, van Montfoort AP. Placentas from pregnancies conceived by IVF/ICSI have a reduced DNA methylation level at the H19 and MEST differentially methylated regions. Human Reproduction. 2013;**28**(4):1117-1126

[62] Ghosh J, Coutifaris C, Sapienza C, Mainigi M. Global DNA methylation levels are altered by modifiable clinical manipulations in assisted reproductive technologies. Clinical Epigenetics. 2017;**9**(1):14

[63] Schoolcraft WB, Treff NR, Stevens JM, Ferry K, Katz-Jaffe M, Scott RT Jr. Live birth outcome with trophectoderm biopsy, blastocyst vitrification, and single-nucleotide polymorphism microarray-based comprehensive chromosome screening in infertile patients. Fertility and Sterility. 2011;**96**:638-640

[64] Bisignano A, Wells D, Harton G, Munne S. PGD and aneuploidy screening for 24 chromosomes: Advantages and disadvantages of competing platforms. Reproductive Biomedicine Online. 2011;**23**:677-685

[65] Wong CC, Loewke KE, Bossert NL, Behr B, De Jonge CJ, Baer TM, et al. Non-invasive imaging of human embryos before embryonic genome activation predicts development to the blastocyst stage. Nature Biotechnology. 2010;**28**:1115-1121

[66] Kirkegaard K, Ahlstrom A, Ingerslev HJ, et al. Choosing the best embryo by time lapse versus standard morphology. Fertility and Sterility. 2015;**103**:323-332

[67] Yang Z, Zhang J, Salem SA, et al. Selection of competent blastocysts for transfer by combining time-lapse monitoring and array CGH testing for patients undergoing preimplantation genetic screening: A prospective study with sibling oocytes. BMC Medical Genomics. 2014;**7**:38

[68] Armstrong S, Arroll N, Cree LM, et al. Time-lapse systems for embryo incubation and assessment in assisted reproduction. Cochrane Database of Systematic Reviews. 2015;**2**:CD011320

[69] Seli E, Robert C, Sirard MA. OMICS in assisted reproduction: Possibilities and pitfalls. Molecular Human Reproduction. 2010;**16**:513-530

[70] Menezo Y, Elder K, Benkhalifa S, Dale B. DNA methylation and gene expression in IVF. Reproductive Biomedicine Online. 2010;**20**:709-710

[71] Nagy ZP, Jones-Colon S, Roos P, Botros L, Greco E, Dasig J, et al. Metabolomic assessment of oocyte viability. Reproductive Biomedicine Online. 2009;**18**:219-225

[72] Tejera A, Herero J, de Los Santos MJ, Garrido N, Ramsing N, Meseguer M. Oxygen consumption is a quality marker for human oocyte competence conditioned by ovarian stimulation regimens. Fertility and Sterility. 2011;**96**:618-623

[73] Evgeni E, Byron A. Human sperm DNA fragmentation and its correlation

with conventional semen parameters. Journal of Reproduction & Infertility. 2014;**15**(1):2-14

[74] Leach M, Aitken R, Sacks G. Sperm DNA fragmentation abnormalities in men from couples with a history of recurrent miscarriage. Australian and New Zealand Journal of Obstetrics and Gynaecology. 2015;**55**:379-373

[75] Gil M, Shalom V, Carreras S. Sperm selection using magnetic activated cell sorting (MACS) in assisted reproduction: A systematic review and meta-analysis. Journal of Assisted Reproduction and Genetics. 2013;**30**(4):479-485

[76] Cheng Y, Feng Y, Jansson L, Sato Y, Deguchi M, Kawamura K, et al. Actin polymerization-enhancing drugs promote ovarian follicle growth mediated by the hippo signaling effector YAP. The FASEB Journal. 2015;**29**(6):2423-2430

[77] Johnson J, Canning J, Kaneko T, Pru JK, Tilly JL. Germline stem cells and follicular renewal in the postnatal mammalian ovary. Nature. 2004;**428**(6979):145-150

[78] Afifi N, Reyad O. Role of mesenchymal stem cell therapy in restoring ovarian function in a rat model of chemotherapy-induced ovarian failure: A histological and immunohistochemical study. The Egyptian Journal of Histology. 2013;**36**:114-126

[79] Hayashi K, Ogushi S, Kurimoto K, et al. Offspring from oocytes derived from in vitro primordial germ cell–like cells in mice. Science. 2012;**338**:971-975

[80] Callejo J, Salvador S, González-Nuñez S, et al. Live birth in a woman without ovaries after autograft of frozen-thawed ovarian tissue combined with growth factors. Journal of Ovarian Research. 2013;**6**:33-36

[81] Smeets HJM. Preventing the transmission of mitochondrial DNA disorders: Selecting the good guys or kicking out the bad guys. Reproductive BioMedicine Online. 2013;**27**:599-610

[82] Amato P, Tachibana M, Sparman M, Mitalipov S. Three-parent in vitro fertilization: Gene replacement for the prevention of inherited mitochondrial diseases. Fertility and Sterility. 2014;**101**(1):31-35

[83] Mitalipov S, Wolf DP. Clinical and ethical implications of mitochondrial gene transfer. Trends in Endocrinology & Metabolism. 2014;**25**(1):5-7

[84] Kawamura K, Cheng Y, Suzuki N, et al. Hippo signaling disruption and Akt stimulation of ovarian follicles for infertility treatment. PNAS. 2013;**110**(43):17474-17479

Chapter 5

Abortions in First Trimester Pregnancy, Management, Treatment

Panagiotis Tsikouras, Theodora Deftereou, Xanthoula Anthoulaki, Anastasia Bothou, Anna Chalkidou, Fotini Gaitatzi, Ioannis Tsirkas, Arsou Chalil Bourazan, Eirini Bampageorgaka, George Stanulov, Elefterios Chatzimichael, Spyridon Michalopoulos, Panagiotis Petsidis, Georgios Iatrakis, Stefanos Zervoudis, Maria Lambropoulou, Werner Rath and Georgios Galazios

Abstract

The miscarriages' investigation should include a familiar history, gynecological examination and a full laboratory testing including hormonal control, as well as karyotype, maternal immune control and thrombophilia testing. If the physician suspects the cause of abortions is chromosomal due to heredity, a special blood test (karyotype) for the pair is recommended. Chromosomal abnormalities are the most common reason for first trimester abortions, and are impossible to be prevented. Based on the above data, abortion and the subsequent possible infertility should not be considered as a personal failure for the woman and the treating physician. Nowadays, medical advancement provides many options combined with psychological support can actually reduce the miscarriages' risk.

Keywords: spontaneous abortions, recurrent abortions, diagnosis, therapy

1. Introduction

Spontaneous abortions are considered as one of the most common complications in pregnancy. Abortion is defined as the ejection of the fetus until the 20th week and is clinically classified based on ultrasound evaluation. Threatened abortion is usually accompanied by vaginal bleeding without affecting the pregnancy. Incomplete miscarriage is described as incomplete passage of conception products. Complete, when all pregnancy products are spontaneously aborted. Septic abortion when endometrial infection coexists. Finally, recurrent abortions that are defined when three consecutive abortions occur before 20th weeks of gestation [1–5].

More than 80% of miscarriages occur up to 12 weeks. The percentage of clinically recognized abortions (appeared after 6th week) is estimated to be 12–15%. More analytically, 2 miscarriages occurred in 5% of women and ≥3 miscarriages in 1–3% of women [1–5]. Recurrent miscarriages consist of a serious problem for women with physical and psychological consequences. Abortions and especially recurrent miscarriages are considered as heterogeneous groups in regard to etiology [1–5]. Two or more causes can coexist, whereas about 50% of cases are characterized as idiopathic as a result of genetic, anatomical, endocrine, genetic, anatomical, endocrine, autoimmune factors or infections exclusion [1–5].

The number of clinically recognized miscarriages to total number of pregnancies is about 10–15%, while the equivalent of early abortions based only on human chorionic gonadotropin (hCG) measurements is actually much higher (50–60%) and interestingly before and after the implantation it is 30% but are not perceived [1, 6–10].

A positive correlation has been identified between the mother's biological age and the incidence rate of spontaneous abortions. So, a progressive increase of 10-fold afterwards the age of 40 is observed compared to younger women aged <35 years [1, 6–10].

Regarding the gestational age in first trimester and the abortion risk, this counts to 4 and 2%, respectively, in 6th and 8th week of gestation [1, 6–10]. The risk of recurrence in the next pregnancy is minor except of cases diagnosed with congenital uterine abnormalities [1, 6–10].

1.1 Recurrent miscarriages

Recurrent miscarriages are defined as three or more consecutive embryos losses weighing under 500 g. According to bibliography we can find different definitions for miscarriages [1, 11, 12]: two or more miscarriages of clinical pregnancies [7]; three or more miscarriages of the first trimester or one or more miscarriages of the second trimester; three or more miscarriages <14 weeks [1, 11, 12]. Frequency appearance is of quite large (1 in every 300 pregnancies).

Recurrent miscarriages (frequency 1–3% among couples of reproductive age) usually occur during the first trimester and relative risk increases with the number of previous miscarriages [1, 11, 12]. Consequently, after the first miscarriage, this risk reaches 24%, after the second one to 26% and after the third it amounts to 32% [1, 11, 12]. About 10–15% of all clinical recognized pregnancies are aborted and the theoretical risk for three consecutive pregnancy losses is 0.34% [1, 11, 12].

Receiving history includes:

- the gestational age of spontaneous abortions
- the certification in the presence of embryonic pole and heart function
- the symptoms related to the antiphospholipid syndrome and family history of automatic abortions

The possibility to predict the risk of recurrence depends on several factors like as maternal age, fetal parental karyotypes gestational age, presence of various maternal laboratory findings [1, 11, 12].

About 80% of abortions occur during the first trimester, 50–60% of them are based on genetic abnormalities. The risk of pregnancy loss is 2–5% after the recognition of heart function, 5% for women who report two miscarriages and finally 1% of women mentioning more than three miscarriages [1, 11, 12].

Investigation of recurrent pregnancy loss (RPL) begins with personal history, followed by laboratory, genetic, hormonal, anatomic, immunologic, thrombophilic factors and infective reasons that can affect pregnancy outcome. It is quite often that 2 or more factors coexist [11–20]. In half of cases, etiology cannot be identified, so it is described as "Recurrent miscarriages of unknown etiology" [1, 11, 16].

2. Clinical examination

During the clinical examination, a gynecological examination and a check for hyperandrogenemia and hyperprolactinemia signs should be done [1, 17].

3. Laboratory check

A laboratory control includes:

- Karyotype in couple
- Hysteroscopy or hysterosalpingography (HSG)
- Anticardiolipins and LA
- Control of progesterone levels in the middle of the luteal phase cycle
- Check the levels of FSH,LH,PRL and testosterone (2–5th day of period)
- TVS (transvaginal ultrasound) [1, 13–20].

It is of great importance in thrombophilia examinations control to include V Leiden factor and prothrombin 20210 mutation [1, 15–20].

4. Anatomical factors

Anatomical abnormalities that can cause miscarriages are typically recognized using hydrosonohysterography (HSG), hysteroscopy, laparoscopy, possible in same cases magnetic resonance and recently three-dimensional ultrasonography.

Congenital anomalies malformations of the female reproductive tract uterine anatomical abnormalities, such as bicornuate uterus or uterine diaphragm, polyps, heart-shaped ultrasound fibroids are results from failure completion of bilateral duct elongation, fusion, septal resorption of müllerian ducts [13–15].

Especially with regard to fibroids, they may block the development of early pregnancy, but their influence on spontaneous abortions is also affected by other factors such as age and hormonal disorders. Müllerian anomalies occurred in 8–10% of women, who had three or more consecutive spontaneous abortions. The fibromuscular tissue in septate uterus is poorly vascularized fibromuscular tissue that is associated with the highest pregnancy loss rate in some studies reporting an average of 65%. Except the above-mentioned abnormality, high frequency for pregnancy loss is noticed in didelphys, bicornuate and unicornuate uterus [13–15].

Intrauterine adhesions (Asherman syndrome) are acquired uterine defect resulting from infection, endometritis and unsuccessful curettage, which is associated with recurrent miscarriage, oligomenorrhea and amenorrhea and bad prognosis.

Recommended treatment in these cases includes balloon catheter, administration of estrogen and progestin medication [1, 16–18].

Uterine cavity abnormalities including submucosal, intramural >40 myomas, polyps are associated to poorly vascularization of endometrium led to failure of implantation, placenta tissue development and contribute to pregnancy loss. Cervical insufficiency is described as an acquired uterine anomaly, which is depending in painless cervical dilatation, effacement and inability of the uterine cervix to retain the amniosac is the commonest reason for abortion in the second trimester [16–18]. Exposure of the embryo in diethylstilbestrol DES and a variety of environmental factors like thalidomide, infectious agents and ionizing radiation affects the uterine morphology by triggering changes in both the location and amount of HOXA/Hoxa expression in the development of Müllerian ducts. No prospective studies exist. The HOXA genes along the Müllerian ducts, influencing the development of Müllerian ducts are: HOXA9 Oviduct, HOXA10, HOXA11 Uterus, HOXA11, HOXA13 Cervix and HOXA13 Upper vagina [1, 19–21].

5. Chromosomal abnormalities

Genetics reasons of recurrent pregnancy loss be subdivided in embryo abnormalities resulting of known parental genetic pathology and embryo aneuploidy in parents to be chromosomally normal A variety of genetic factors including aneuploidy (gain or loss of a chromosomal), chromosomal imbalance resulting from harbored translocations, inversions, deletions, duplications within chromosomes, single gene mutations led to recurrent pregnancy loss (RPL) [1, 22–33]. In 3–5% of couples with RPL, the ratio of parental chromosome abnormalities in contrast to the general population is 0.7%. The most common chromosomal abnormalities leading to RPL are balanced translocations. The first chromosomally abnormal abortion was reported in 1961. Chromosomal abnormality is approximately responsible for half of the clinically diagnosed abortions in the first trimester. About 50% of them are autosomal trisomy, 20% monosomy XO, 20% polyploidy and 10% variety of other abnormalities [33–35].

5.1 Karyotype examinations in aborted fetus

- Karyotype in couple
- No need for molecular karyotype
- No need for microdeletions control

About 25% of cases exist in the first trimester, in which although the embryos are normal and euploid, they cannot develop properly. The reasons include women with müllerian agenesis and other significant anatomic abnormalities. In the second trimester, the abortion incidence due to a chromosomal abnormality is <20%. Structural chromosome abnormalities (Robertson-type balancing and translocations).

X-inactivation chromosome (?)

aneuploidy of spermatozoa (?).

Recurrent abortion (RA) as well as repeated IVF failure (RIF) has a common underlying factor which is the significant increase in the rate of chromosomal abnormality [35]. The results also suggest that in women with recurrent abortions, the transfer of normal embryos improves the pregnancy rate and live-birth rate in both younger and older women. In these cases, preimplantation genetic diagnosis is recommended, testing for structural chromosomal aberrations like translocations, inversions, removing cells from the resultant embryo or oocyte evaluating the cells for genetic abnormalities and determine the optimal embryos for uterine transfer [35–37]. Last year, novel technologies like microarrays, fluorescence in situ hybridization and biopsy of embryo blastocyst are widely used [34–36].

5.2 Lifestyle and environment

Women with RPL have reproductive difficulties because they are concerned about various toxins and agents within the environment. It is of great importance to counseling these couples in health care institutions to have current and accurate information and to avoid exposures to these substances [37, 38]. The rate of spontaneous abortion is positively associated to cigarette smoking, alcohol consumption, obesity, body mass index (BMI, weight in kilograms divided by square of height in meters) >30 kg/m^2, caffeine intake (excess of 300 mg/day) and ionizing radiation [37, 38].

6. Immunological factors

In some case, a failure to activate a normal control mechanism to prevent an immune reaction against self is observed and this subsequently led to autoimmune response. Natural killer cells are attached to the cytotrophoblast of the embryo. However, the mechanism by which such cells may or may not affect the embryo is not proven. When implantation occurs, there is a slight inflammatory response. Patient with infertility and recurrent miscarriages develop less prominent reaction that may prevent the embryo from implanting [39, 40]. Autoimmune abortions are thought to be caused by the presence of autoantibodies that already exist in the woman against membrane phospholipids, thyroid antigens, nuclear antigens, syncytiotrophoblast cells or against other organelles or tissues [39, 40].

About 10–15% of all women have antinuclear antibodies regardless of medical history of RPL. In cases of presence of antinuclear antibodies, the possibility of successful pregnancy outcome is independent of antibodies existence [39, 40].

Autoimmune factors causing RPL are: antiphospholipid antibody syndrome, aPL antibodies (anticardiolipin antibodies and lupus anticoagulant), ß2 glycoprotein antibodies, phosphatidyl serine. Antibody hemeostasis in systemic circulation is different between men and women, just because women need to be better equipped, so that they can cope with the required immune tolerance in fetal antigens derived from them [39, 40].

The “thermostat” is therefore positioned higher in women, as a result, autoimmune diseases have much higher incidence in women. If autoantibodies are found in relation to a pathological condition, this means: whether they are the pathogenetic factors of the disease (autoimmune hemolytic anemia); whether it is the result of a previous pathological process (autoantibodies against cardiac muscle after its destruction) and whether they are causative agents without damaging themselves, which is the most common, as is believed [40, 41].

If the antibodies are present in the mother’s serum as a result of allogeneic stimulation during pregnancy, then they are not considered to be autoantibodies unless they exist previously [40, 41]. Until now, there is no common point of the effect of pregnancy on the production of autoantibodies. Although no clear increase in autoantibodies has been found during normal pregnancy, an increase in some of them has been reported in pathological pregnancies, most of which have been described as antiphospholipid antibodies [40, 41]. In the group of recurrent miscarriages, 15% were certified positive findings for the lupus anticoagulant or antiphospholipid antibodies or both of them. It is important to notice that lupus anticoagulant is not synonymous with systemic lupus erythematosus (SLE), where it is found in only 5–15% [40, 41].

6.1 Antiphospholipid antibodies

Antiphospholipid antibodies (APAs) are a family of immunoglobulins which react with anions of phospholipids or anions of phospholipid-protein complexes in the cell membrane of the syncytiotrophoblast [1, 41, 42].

The finding of aPL antibodies is associated to adverse pregnancy outcomes such inducing vessel thrombosis of the surrounding placental maternal unit, placenta infarction, and fetal death. The primary mechanism in the first trimester depends on a deleterious effect directly on trophoblastic cells, inhibition of secretion of human placental chorionic gonadotropin, and the expression of trophoblast cell adhesion molecules (a1, a5 integrins, E, VE-cadherins). The most widely used are anti-cardiolipin (diphosphatidyl-glycerol) [1, 41, 42].

Others are anti-phosphatidylserine anti-phosphatidylethanolamine, anti-phosphatidylcholine, anti-phosphatidylinositol, and phosphatidic acid. Large variation in APHA measurements between laboratories and in the same laboratory for the same patient and great fluctuation in the values during pregnancy are observed.

It is questionable whether the same or other substnces (anti-β2-glycoprotein I) have similar impact according to recurrent pregnancy loss [42–45].

Possible action of APAs on miscarriages:

Abnormalities in endothelial cell function of vessels (decrease in production of arachidonic acid prostacyclin and a relative increase of thromboxane which is a potent vasoconstrictor and promotes platelet aggregation).

Obstructive angiopathy (reaction with anion phospholipids exposed after vessel damage).

Platelet stimulation and/or adhesion (in damaged platelets, APAs bind phosphatidylserine to the structural element of the inner membrane of the platelets and promote platelet aggregation and thrombus formation).

Placental infarction (microscopic arterial thrombosis and necrotic fibrous deposition have been found). It also appears to be due to reduced flow in the vessels, as has been found to occur in the umbilical and maternal arteries in patients with lupus or APS. This situation resembles a destruction of the vessels through antibodies after heart transplantation, coronary bypass, or angioplasty [42–45].

Inhibition of protein C stimulation in S. These two proteins, after their activation, inactivate clotting factors Va and VIIa. Stimulating their stimulation creates an increased tendency for coagulation.

Reduction of levels of annexin V, a protein with potent antithrombotic effect on the surface between trophoblast and endothelial cells.

Effect on placental function: (ACA inhibits the secretion of gonadotropin secretion from placenta, which can act on the secretion of hormones from the placenta, negatively affecting the viability of the fetus).

Phospholipids bind to the surface of trophoblast, and this results in direct destruction of cells, inhibition of syncytia formation, decrease of hCG production and defective penetration into maternal peristalsis.

6.2 Autoimmune factors

Antiphospholipid syndrome: high levels of antiphospholipid antibodies and history of miscarriages and/or endometrial death and/or thrombosis—risk of autoimmune in subsequent pregnancy ~90% [46, 47].

6.3 Clinical criteria

Vascular thrombosis (one or more clinical episodes of venous, arterial, or small vessel thrombosis in any tissue or organ).

Gestational complications (one or more recurrent miscarriages after the 10th week of gestation, one or more preterm births and one or more recurrent miscarriages before the 10th week of gestation).

Laboratory criteria: cardiolipin antibodies (IgG or IgM anti-cardiolipins, at moderate or high levels in two or more measurements over a period of at least 6 weeks between them).

Lupus anticoagulant (in two or more measurements at least 6 weeks apart) [44–47].

7. Antiphospholipid syndrome: management

Steroids (complications: pregnancy and prematurity) are not recommend based on current publication evidence. It is reported that the maternal and fetal complications increase without affecting the pregnancy outcome and live births [43–47].

7.1 Prednisolone, between 10 and 20 mg daily dosage

It may prevent recycling in the circulation of cardiolipins or suspend the discharge of embryo toxic factors or factors associated with HLA. In addition, it lowers NK (CD56+/CD16+) cell percentage. It has been associated with pregnancy hypertension, diabetes mellitus, and mainly with premature labor and low-weight new-born babies. Aspirin should be given preconceptually. **Aspirin in low dosage** (80–100 mg daily) may suspend cyclooxygenase (COX) action on platelets, by suspending the composition of thromboxane thrombosis and thus preventing vascular thrombosis in placental blood vessels. At discontinuance after around 32 weeks, heparin (does not pass the placenta) should be started after the first positive pregnancy test and should be continued until of labor to avoid thrombosis risk: hypo-heparin, for example, **heparin of low molecular weight,** one injection daily. Anticoagulant action (reinforces the action of antithrombin III), while it may bind AFAs, thus prevents chorionic villus sampling (CVS) phospholipids from being destroyed, by assisting in the successful implantation in the early stages of pregnancy [43–47]. Thrombocytopenia and osteoporosis check-up. Discontinuation after 34 weeks of pregnancy and prior to giving birth. **(Now in labor)**.

It appears that combining aspirin and heparin has the best results. Patients should start taking heparin as early as possible when pregnant and continue until labor and during puerperium [42–50]. Combination of aspirin and heparin is associated with better results. Heparin subcutaneously, for example, low molecular weight heparin one injection per day may prevent recycling of circulating anti-cardiolipins or suppress the secretion of embryotoxic agents or HLA-related agents. It also reduces the percentage of NK (CD56+/CD16+) cells [46–50]. It has been associated with gestational hypertension and diabetes mellitus and mainly with premature labor and low birth weight neonates. Combination of aspirin with heparin, aspirin with prednisolone, or all three is associated to satisfactory results. It seems that the combination of aspirin and heparin works best. Heparin should be started as soon as possible in pregnancy and should be maintained until the labor and postpartum especially when the risk of thrombosis is high [42–50]. Intravenous immunoglobulin therapy IVIG (no superior to the combination of aspirin and heparin) Intravenous injection of high doses of gamma globulin (300–500 mg/kg body weight). An increase inT-immunosuppressive cells, decreases the activity of natural killer cells, inhibition of transport by the mother's placenta of IgG, inhibition of Fc receptors in macrophages and, especially, multivalent immunosuppression. To avoid the adverse reactions of heparin therapy, it is recommended to add calcium 600 mg twice daily and vitamin D supplementation 400 IU daily to decrease the osteoporosis risk. The platelet count should be weekly examined in the first two weeks after treatment with heparin because bleeding could occur due to heparin induced thrombocytopenia [42–50].

8. Endocrine factors

Mentioned here are polycystic ovary syndrome (PCOS) due to high levels of luteinizing hormone (LH), corpus luteum (CL) deficiency, nonregulated diabetes mellitus during conception period, thyroid malfunction, thrombophilic factors, alloimmunological factors: PCOS, menstrual complications, hypertrichosis, polycystic ovaries, and resistance to insulin. The contribution of endocrinological factor as reasons of RPL including luteal phase deficiency, untreated hypothyroidism, abnormal glucose metabolism hyperprolactinemia, and diminished ovarian reserve is average by 8–12% [51–54].

8.1 Corpus luteum deficiency

Corpus luteum malfunction association with RPLs still remains a hypothesis, despite the fact that there are studies that reveal that it is responsible for 12–28% of cases. Luteal phase deficiency is defined as an inability of the corpus luteum to secrete progesterone either in increased satisfactory amounts or for too short duration. This inability to function is established by alteration of preovulatory estrogen stimulation, which led to poor oocyte quality and a poorly functioning corpus luteum. The diagnosis should be confirmed either with endometrial biopsy which is not recommended as diagnostic modality or if serum progesterone levels are <10 ng/ml [51–54]. Strategy of treatments of corpus luteum malfunction has a wide variation and includes administration of progesterone or human chorionic gonadotropin induction or a combination of these. Progesterone administration either as intravaginal suppositories 50–100 mg or as intramuscular injections 50 mg IM is considered necessary only within RCTs [51–54].

8.2 Hyperprolactinemia

Hyperprolactinemia is an endocrinopathy which led to infertility and abortions due to anovulation. It is not clear whether it is associated with RPLs. Increased prolactin levels interact with the hypothalamic pituitary ovarian axis, reducing the folliculogenesis or leading to a small duration of luteal phase. Studies reveal that it affects progesterone discharge at luteal stage; however, this situation has not been confirmed in humans. A randomized control trial including 64 hyperprolactinemic women with RPL treated with bromocriptine was associated with a higher rate of successful pregnancy, whereas PRL levels were significantly higher in women that miscarried (85.7 vs. 52.4%) [55–58].

8.3 Dopamine agonists

Currently, there is no sufficient evidence for effectiveness of dopamine agonist evaluation in preventing future miscarriage in women with idiopathic hyperprolactinemia and a history of recurrent miscarriage [55–57].

8.4 Diabetes mellitus

Women with nonregulated DM I: diabetes mellitus (DM) in women with RPLs is associated with a higher incidence of spontaneous abortions in relation to women with euglycemic metabolism preconceptually. A well controlled diabetes mellitus decreases the rates of recurrent pregnancy loss. Testing for fasting insulin and glucose and hemoglobin A1c usually have an increased modality for the evaluation of insulin resistance. The metformin administration seems to improve pregnancy outcome and is it safe in the first trimester [55–57].

8.5 Thyroid gland disorders

It is well known that hypothyroidism without therapy increases the risk of abortion. Treatment before attempting a pregnancy is clearly recommend as well as keeping a TSH level between 1.0–2.5 UIU/ml in the first trimester. In cases with TSH levels higher than 2.5 MIU/ml, levothyroxine should be started at a minimum dose of 50 μg/d.

Anti-thyroid Abs is associated with RPLs when detected before the start of pregnancy or at an early stage.

Hypothyroidism is involved with obstetric complications like infertility, abortions, anemia, preeclampsia, placental abruption, fetal death, preterm birth, and low birth weight [55–58].

8.6 Alloimmune dysfunction

- Elevated CD56+ lymphocyte levels

- Increased NK cell levels in the secretory phase of endometrium

- Higher levels in NK cells during the endometrium secretory phase. Strong association between maternal type Th2-cell immunity and successful pregnancy outcome. Recurrent abortions: associated with immunity type Th1 (lF-γ, TNF, lL-12, 58)

8.7 Diminished ovarian reserve

Increased levels of FSH in the early follicular phase of menstrual cycle are significant for diminished ovarian reserve. In the least years, another marker antimüllerian hormone is better to identify the number of follicular units for recruitment. It is recommended that women with RPL visit healthcare services to have appropriate counselling to treat endocrinological disorders [59].

8.8 PCOS

Polycystic ovary syndrome (PCOS) is associated with increased frequency of RPL and has an uncertain prevalence, because factors associated with PCOS such as obesity, insulin resistance, LH rise, and hyperandrogenemia may be the reason and not PCOS as a whole [60–68]. The incidence of abortions in spontaneous ovulation is difficult to determine. Diagnostic criteria for this heterogeneous disorder have not been present in the past. Hypersecretion of LH and elevate androgen levels possibly led to RPL [60–68]. The association of excess androgens and RPL is not clear. The hyperinsulinemia in PCOS that is a consequence of insulin resistance involving plasminogen activator inhibitor-1(PAI-1) which inhibits plasminogen activation and subsequent fibrinolysis, has potential thromboembolic effect that makes women with PCOS in high risk for recurrent pregnancy loss [60–68].

8.9 Why LH rise may result in abortion

- premature oocyte maturation
- hyperandrogenemia may impact on oocytes
- high androgens may affect endometrium

8.10 Role of androgen abortion

- androgens may affect endometrium
- in vitro studies show inhibitory effect of androstenedione
- in endometrial cell growth and activity (glycodelin secretion)
- glycodelin inhibits endometrial immune response to the embryo [60–68]

8.11 Endometrium

- gene hoxa10 is thought to be essential for implantation.
- the expression of this gene is decreased when testosterone is elevated.

8.12 Hyperinsulinemia: abortion

Preimplantation environment is affected by decreasing:

1. expression of glycodelin—which inhibits endometrial immune response to the embryo and
2. IGF—binding protein-1, which facilitates adhesion progress at the fetomaternal interface. Plasma plasminogen activator inhibitor-1 concentrations are increased in hyperinsulinemia leading to hypofibrinolytic state and thrombophilia [60–68]

8.13 PCO—abortion: thrombophilia

Plasminogen activator inhibitor gene (PAI-1) activity (i.e., hypofibrinolysis) is elevated in PCO.

Metformin reduces gene activity from 42.5 to 12.4 U/ml, that is, correct tendency for thrombosis which improves uteroplacental flow.

9. Metformin treatment

PAI-1 activity fell 44% in women with live births.
PAI-1 activity increased 19% in women with abortion.

10. Pregnancy loss and possible beneficial effects of metformin

1. Decreased levels of androgen may improve endometrial function; IR resistance is decreased

2. Glycodelin and IGF-1 protein expression is corrected

3. Glycodelin inhibits endometrial immune response to the embryo

4. IGF-1 improves the adhesion process at the fetomaternal interface

5. Hypofibrinolytic activity is reduced by decreased PAI-1 activity (which induces hypofibrinolytic activity) [60–68].

11. The prevalence of abortion in PCO is probably elevated

1. Obesity very probably implicated

2. Insulin resistance probably but may INDIRECTLY affect the parameters which are influenced by metformin

3. The role of LH needs to be elucidated

4. Endometrial factor probable

5. Oocyte factor probable

6. PAI-1 factor probable

7. Further prospective studies needed to elucidate the significance of these factors

Usually, women with PCOS require different treatments due to variety of reasons so we can use metformin, diet and infertility drugs. Therapeutic management combines normalization of weight and administration of metformin to reduce mainly the RPL rate [60–68].

12. Infections

Any infection with high fever can lead to miscarriage rubella virus, cytomegalovirus passing the placenta and affecting the fetus, malaria, mycoplasma, and trypanosomiasis.

Several studies have confirmed the role of infections as a cause of miscarriage especially in the second trimester of pregnancy; however, their role in the first trimester miscarriages remains unclear [69–74].

12.1 Infective factors' mechanisms of action

Toxic metabolic bio-products, endotoxins, exotoxins, or cytokines may have a direct effect on the uterus and the fetoplacental unit chronic endometrial infection following after lineal infection (M. hominis, Chlamydia, Ureaplasma urealyticum, and HSV) may affect the fetus implantation. Fetal infections are possible to cause fetal death or severe malformations incompatible with fetal livability (rubella, parvovirus B19, CMV, HSV, and syphilis). Placental infection probably causes placental deficiency with consequent fetal death. Amnionitis in the first trimester may have a similar effect on chorioamnionitis in the third trimester (causing premature labor). Various microorganisms with such effect, as L. monocytogenes, are suspected [69–74].

12.2 Correlation between the various supposed mechanisms of automatic abortions and specific infectious factors

Mechanisms:

1. Embryotoxicity

2. Placental deficiency

3. Endometritis/endocervicitis

4. Amnionitis

Microorganisms: rubella, parvovirus B19, CMV, HSV, syphilis, Chlamydia, Mycoplasma, Ureaplasma, and various Gram-positive or Gram-negative bacteria (*L. monocytogenes*).

None of the above-mentioned infectious agents are usually confirmed to lead to RPL. Each high fever infection may lead to pregnancy loss. Viruses such as rubella and cytomegalovirus infection (CMV) go through the placenta and affect the embryo, as well as lead to malaria, chlamydia, mycoplasma, and trypanosomiasis [69–74].

Quite a few studies have confirmed that infections are to blame when it comes to miscarriages, especially during the second trimester of pregnancy; however, their role in the first trimester miscarriages remains unspecified.

12.3 Recurrent miscarriages of unknown etiology

New techniques in molecular biology and genetics could recognize the importance of "locality" for mutations. Detection of new mutations in immunological and other molecules is involved in the pathophysiology of abortions. It is of great importance to immediately start appropriate antibiotic therapy based on a test of cure culture, when cervical and vaginal infections are identified and to extend the treatment for both parents [75, 76].

12.4 Thrombophilia

Pregnancy is a condition that predisposes to hypercoagulation. The pregnant woman is in a state of increased tendency for coagulation (hypercoagulable state). The action of the fibrinolytic system decreases during pregnancy, particularly in the placenta, mainly due to an increase in inhibitors of the plasminogen activator [77–84].

Pregnancy and coagulation mechanisms include the following:

- Increase of coagulation precursors **(procoagulant factors)**
- Decrease in levels of physiologically existing anticoagulant factors (**naturally occurring anticoagulants**)
- Reduction of fibrinogenolysis
- "Modified" maternal response to hemostasis (**'disordered' maternal hemostatic response)** [77–84]

Correlation not quite clear!

Pregnancy is a state of hypercoagulation (hypercoagulable state). This hypercoagulable state do not necessarily causes thrombosis and the miscarriage is not due to thrombosis.and a lot of patients with miscarriages. This predisposition for thrombosis may lead to malfunction in the fetoplacental unit. A disorder in the balance between activators and inhibitors of plasminogen can lead to defective placentation [77–84]. The infiltration of trophoblast in arcuate arteries is essential for implantation, placentation, and consequently a regular continuation of pregnancy. Defective penetration is a common pathological finding in placenta preparations by women with excretion and also preeclampsia or intrauterine fetal growth delay [77–84].

Placenta abnormalities include excessive implantation and placenta accreta.

Increasing thrombophilic factors and five more frequent thrombophilic polymorphisms: a) V Leiden factor; b) MHTHFRC 677T; c) MTHFRA1298C; d) Factor VA1299H; and e) factor II G20210A are predisposition to venous thromboembolism (VTE). None of the five thrombophilic mutations, alone or in combination, was found to significantly increase the risk of miscarriages [77–84].

12.5 Thrombophilic factors

V Leiden: women with RPLs and V Leiden mutation: there is no discrimination test for those who will have recurrent miscarriages from those that have a term pregnancy.

Treatment: prophylactic administration of heparin without the confirmation of RCT is prescribed for known mutations of the factor V Leiden and also for the cases that there is indication of placental thrombosis [77–84].

C677T MTHFR polymorphism: previous studies have shown conflicting results between the MTHFR C677T genotype and the recurrent miscarriages.

5,10-methylentetrahydrofolate reductase catalyzes the conversion of 5,10-methylentetrahydrofolic acid to 5-methyltetrahydrofolic acid.

5-methyltetrahydrofolic acid takes part in the methylation of homocysteine in methionine.

Substitution of a cytosine molecule by a thymine molecule at position 677 increases the incidence of homocysteine and thrombophilia.

The reduced activity of MTHFR and hyperhomocysteinemia is clinically manifested when lack of folic acid coexists [77–84].

Treatment: administration of 0.5–2 mg of folic acid leads to homocysteine normal levels [77–84].

12.6 Combination of multiple mild thrombophilic factors

12.6.1 Plasminogen activator inhibitor (PAI)

Increased activity of PAI: genetic factors, metabolic disorders of insulin resistance syndrome, hypertension, smoking, etc.

PAI-1: the major physiological inhibitor of plasminogen activation plays a central role in fibrinolysis.

PAI-2: trophoblast and macrophages. Increased PAI activity has been linked to recurrent miscarriages.

4G polymorphism of PAI-1 gene is associated with high levels of PAI-1 and reduced fibrinolytic activity.

Homozygous for 4G has been complicated with preeclampsia, prematurity, IUGR, and placental ablation.

12.7 Combining multiple subtle thrombophilic factors

12.7.1 Factor XII deficiency (Hagemann)

- low molecular weight heparin (LMWH)
- heparin
- LMWH vs. heparin
- one injection per day
- anti-Xa follow-up is not necessary
- decreased risk of osteoporosis
- reduced risk of thrombocytopenia
- safe for the fetus as it does not pass the placenta
- more likely outcome in obstetric complications [77–84]

12.8 Increase of homocysteine and thrombophilia

As mentioned before, decreased MTHFR activity and hyperhomocysteinemia are only obvious as long as there is folic acid deficiency. Substitution with folic acid prevents any phenotypic expression of C677T polymorphism.

Prediction for women with polymorphism who are going to have a spontaneous abortion [77–84]:

Treatment: the administration of 0.5–2 mg folic acid reduces homocysteine levels to normal [77–84].

Homocysteine: homocysteine is an amino acid formed as an intermediate of metabolism of methionine. Elevated blood levels of homocysteine (hyperhomocysteinemia) consist an important cardiovascular risk factor, which in recent years have significance similar to hypercholesterolemia [85–90].

The detection of women with congenital hyperthyroidism that have much more frequent complications in gestation has led to an investigation of the association between homocysteine and pregnancy complications associated with placental vascular lesions such as placental abruption, preeclampsia, abortions, fetal death, and restriction of intrauterine fetal growth. Hyperhomocysteinemia is also associated with spinal tube deficits due to folic acid insufficiency. The result that women with hyperhomocysteinemia of relative cause show complications much more frequently has led to the investigation of obstetric complications with homocysteine, which are relevant with vascular placental failure such as placental abruption, pre-eclampsia, recurrent miscarriages, stillbirth, and intrauterine growth restriction [85–90].

Methionine consist of an important amino-acid that participates in cell growth and division by providing methyl groups in the biosynthesis of t-RNA, DNA, and proteins. Methionine constitutes a necessary amino acid that plays a crucial role in cellular increase and division by providing methyl groups to t-RNA, DNA, and protein biosynthesis. Homocysteine is synthesized after a methyl group transposition from methionine. The 50% could be catalyzed with a sulfureted group transposition into cystathionine. The remaining 50% of homocysteine may be reformed to methionine by removing a methyl group from two sources: (1) the metabolism of tetrahydrofolic acid (THF) and (2) the catabolism of betaine. Three enzymes take part in these metabolic pathways: methionine synthetase (MS), cysteine synthetase (CBS), and methyl-tetrahydrofolic acid reductase (MTHFR). Vitamin B6 (pyridoxine) consists of a coenzyme in the CBS and MTHFR function, while B12 is a coenzyme in the MS function. The adequacy of folic acid is necessary for both functions. The vascular endothelium may only produce CBS and MTHFR, rendering it more sensitive to disturbances in homocysteine metabolism [85–90].

Homocysteine levels >15–16 μmol/l in nonpregnant women and >6–8 μmol/l in the third trimester of pregnancy are considered abnormal. In pregnancy, homocysteine levels decrease progressively and reach a minimum in the second trimester, while increasing slightly in the third trimester. Causes of fluctuations are estrogen, blood dilution, and increased metabolism of homocysteine in the liver, as well as its removal to the fetus. Mild disturbances in homocysteine metabolism can be detected if its levels are measured 6 hours after methionine administration. In this case, levels >51 μmol/l are considered pathologically out of pregnancy, but for pregnancy, there are no measurements [85–90].

Generally, the increase in basal levels of homocysteine represents deficits in remethylation, whereas the increase in homocysteine after methionine loading reveals deficiencies related to the transfer of the sulfur group.

Hyperhomocysteinemia may be related to mutations in genes controlling the production of CBS and MHTFR and environmental factors such as B6, B12, and folic acid deficiency. Drugs that interfere with the metabolism or absorption of these vitamins, decreased homocysteine excretion in chronic renal failure, and other causes (hypothyroidism, hepatic failure, malignant anemia, and cancer) cause hypercholesterolemia [85–90].

It is worth highlighting cases with genetic mutations of the enzymes that cause hyperomyeloidemia, because they are common and appear to play a role in the course of pregnancy [85–90].

12.9 Laboratory criteria

Antibodies vs. cardiolipins: anti-cardiolipins lgG or lgM, in medium or high levels in 2 or more cases, with a time distance of at least 6 weeks between them.

Lupusanticoagulant: in two or more cases with a time distance of at least weeks between them.

- Antiphospholipid antibodies

- Acute infections
- Medicine (chlorpromazine and hydralazine)
- Chronic infections (syphilis and hepatitis C)
- No thrombotic effects
- Antiphospholipid syndrome
- Recurrent abortions
- Endometrial death
- Pre-eclampsia
- IUGR
- B2 glycoprotein 1
- Annexin-V: a protein with strong, anticoagulant action.
- Multiple placental micro-thrombosis [85–90].

13. Pregnancy and hyperhomocysteinemia

The existence of high homocysteine levels in the blood has a harmful effect on the placenta and decidua and is associated with the appearance of recurrent abortion and placental abruption. Hyperhomocysteinemia has been found to cause more complications such as pre-eclampsia, stillbirth, and deceleration of intrauterine growth [85–90].

13.1 Hyperhomocysteinemia and spinal tube deficiency

Hyperhomocysteinemia and spinal tube deficiency (NTD) are associated with insufficient MS and MFTHR function, leading to homocysteine accumulation. Reduced methionine methylation and methyl group (necessary for myelin creation) deficiency are responsible for the above complications and not homocysteine effects [10]. Low folic acid levels or reduced intake in cases with increased need (heat sensitive MTHFR) are responsible for spinal tube deficiencies, but also homocysteine level increase. Hyperhomocysteinemia has also been associated with congenital abnormalities on the face and body. Administering 500 mg folic acid for 4 weeks prior to conception or even at the first stage of pregnancy has been found to reduce homocysteine levels by 22% [90–95].

The gene C677T and MTHFR frequency combined with the dietary habits of a population are the reason for variety in NTD appearance in different populations. In Holland, homozygous C677T of MTHFR polymorphism carriers is at 10–16% NTD risk compared to 5% of witnesses. A1298C, a second type of polymorphism, was discovered with just as high risk NTD levels in case of homozygosity [90–95].

13.2 Hyperhomocysteinemia and pre-eclampsia

Several researchers compared patient groups with witnesses, found an increased hyperhomocysteinemia frequency, as well as increased C677T of MTHFR mutation frequency in women with pre-eclampsia. So, they were led to the conclusion that it may also constitute a genetic factor in pre-eclampsia manifestation [90–95].

In large woman study groups where homocysteine levels were evaluated in the second trimester of gestation either prospectively or recursively, it was found that the relevant pre-eclampsia risk in women with hyperhomocysteinemia was between 1.32 and 3.2%, while in primigravida, it reached 9.7% and in those who were obese, it reached 6.9%. Certainly, patient choice (with heavy, premature pre-eclampsia) has a lot to do with the various levels of pre-eclampsia in incidence of appearance of hyperhomocysteinemia in the bibliography. In a prospective study of 1049 pregnant women, at their 16th week of gestation, homocysteine levels did not appear to be different amongst patients with an uncomplicated course of gestation and those with pre-eclampsia. It is undetermined whether homocysteine levels should be evaluated in all women with a history of serious pre-eclampsia in a previous pregnancy. Repeated studies in women with angiopathy and high homocysteine levels have proved that pre-eclampsia was seven times more frequent in their pregnancies when compared to those with normal homocysteine levels. Homocysteine does not appear to activate the endothelium as there was not found a comparison between fibronectin and homocysteine during the episode of pre-eclampsia. A study revealed that administration of folic acid and vitamins in women with a history of heavy early course pre-eclampsia decreases its frequency and severity in the subsequent pregnancy, but because these studies were quite small and not random, other greater ones are in progress. At the moment, no specific genotype has been associated with more severe or premature types of the disease. Therefore, homozygosity in C677T had an applicable pre-eclampsia risk of 2.6% (95% CI 1.4–5.1) and a hyperhomocysteinemia risk of 20.6% (95% CI 3.6–121.6) [90–95].

13.3 Hyperhomocysteinemia and recurrent abortions

High homocysteine levels have proven to be embryo toxic in guinea pigs through the vascular decidua and villi network destruction. Steegers-Theunissen and Co. found that between 8th and 12th week of pregnancy, there are high methionine levels and low homocysteine levels in the extra-embryonic cavity and amniotic fluid compared to the mother, suggesting that homocysteine accumulation may be toxic. Increased miscarriages in the first trimester are not linked to angiopathy, but to methyl group deficiency and defective DNA composition. Wouters and Co. were the first to notice the high hyper-homocysteinemia frequency in the 14% of cases with recurrent abortion with no prior normal pregnancies and in 33% of those with a history of normal pregnancy. Another study in 100 patients with a history of consecutive spontaneous abortions found homocysteinaemia in 12% of them, C677T of MTHFR mutation in 20%, and decreased folic acid levels in 15% of patients. Supplementation of high levels (15 mg) of folic acid and vitamin B6 (750 mg) to 28 patients with recurrent abortion cases improved homocysteine levels and the 17 pregnancies that followed had a successful outcome. In an after-analysis, homocysteine presence with or without methionine loading showed an increased hyper-homocysteinaemia risk by 4.2 and 2.7%, respectively. In another study where MTHFR genotypes were sought after in embryonic tissues and newborns, all genotype associations were found in embryonic tissue, while in newborns, there were no combinations of three or more mutant alleles. This reveals that embryos with a lot of mutations may be miscarried. As a result, it is proved that there is a correlation between homocysteine metabolic disorder and habitual abortions, but it is not clear whether administering vitamins before conception may prevent them [95–100].

13.4 Hyperhomocysteinemia and placental abruption

Placental biopsy in cases with abruption shows vasculopathy compatible with stenosis, necrosis, thrombosis, and atherosclerosis in the spinal arteries. Homocysteine in blood vessels acts by removing the methyl groups necessary for the DNA composition of multiplying cells. In many studies, hyperhomocysteinemia has been linked to placental abruption. In an after-analysis, folic acid deficiency was found to increase placental abruption frequency by 25.9% (95% CI-736.3) and hyperhomocysteinemia by 5.3% (95% CI 1.8–15.9). The presence of C677T of MTHFR polymorphism increases placental angiopathy risk by 2.45% (95% CI 1.00–6.02). In placental angiopathy cases, endothelium proteins are released in the blood, such as the von Willebrand factor (vWF), the activator of plasma tissue tPA (tissue plasma activator), the inhibitor of this activator PAI-1 (plasma activator inhibitor-1), fibronectin, and thrombomodulin that act as malfunction indicators. Women with hyperhomocysteinemia appeared to have a disproportionate tPA/PAI-1 ratio and a high vWF, while women with a placental abruption history had a high vWF and thrombomodulin. Thrombomodulin levels were in proportion with homocysteine levels. Administering antioxidant vitamins (folic acid, pyridoxine, and hydroxocobalamin) reduced the tPA/PAI-1 ratio but did not affect vWF, while the sole administration of folic acid reduced vWF levels. Combining hyperhomocysteinemia with thrombophilia, increases placental abruption risk by 3.4 [95–100].

Finally, angiopathy resulting from hyperhomocysteinemia may be at least theoretically involved in placental abruption, therefore it may be useful for cases with abruption in the future to be checked for thrombophilia and hyperhomocysteinemia and receive antioxidant vitamin treatment [95–100].

13.5 Other cases of hyperhomocysteinemia effects during pregnancy

Hyperhomocysteinemia may be associated with increased endometrial death by different mechanisms such as congenital disorders and pre-eclampsia, but its significance as an independent factor is in question. In a small group of patients, it was found to coexist with 11% frequency, while in a different group it was no more apparent than the rest of the population. The findings for its role in slowing intrauterine growth are contradictory. In another group of patients, hyperhomocysteinemia levels were as high as 38% and in a different group that was checked after methionine loading in women with a history of slowing intrauterine growth, hyperhomocysteinemia levels reached 19.2%. On the contrary, in a recursive review of the course of pregnancy in women who were CBS mutation carriers, newborns did not appear to have lower birth weight [95–100].

14. Hyperhomocysteinemia treatment

Treatment with vitamin B6, B12, and folic acid on its own or combined with other vitamins has been evaluated on small groups of patients with coronary artery disease and obstetrical complications and has been found to induce homocysteine levels and incidents by 30–50% in these groups. In other studies, vitamin C and E were given as antioxidant factors. The significance of adding aspirin or heparin in these groups still remains questionable, even though we can conclude that normalizing homocysteine levels should be enough, in order to achieve the therapeutic response. From the above-mentioned factors, we can estimate that even if there is no unanimity, it is within reason to check homocysteine levels in cases with a history of NTD, pre-eclampsia, recurrent abortions, and perhaps in cases with placental abruption and endometrial death. It is valuable to look further into the results from administering vitamins in these cases [95–100].

15. Further investigations

We and other researchers have been searching for such predictive blood biomarkers of miscarriage. Macrophage inhibitory cytokine 1 (MIC-1), which is During the first trimester of gestation macrophage inhibitory cytokine 1 (MIC-1), which is presented in the syncytiotrophoblast and deciduas increases in serum and it is proposed to play an immunomodulatory role in the progression of the pregnancy. Pregnancy is considered as an ideal condition to study the regulation mechanisms of vascular growth under physiologic circumstances. Fetal vasculogenesis, angiogenesis, and vascular adaptation of the uterine circulation are one of a kind [101–104]. There is strong evidence bracing a close relationship between embryonic development and the state of vascularization of the chorionic villi. Normal chorionic villous vascularization is crucial for the normal development of pregnancy. However, it is not well known whether abnormal changes in utero-placental vascular development predispose to abortions [101–104]. The development of a normal functioning placental vascular network requires an important degree of coordination between various angiogenic and angiostatic factors and is exquisitely dependent on signals exchanged between these factors. Abnormalities in the development of placental vasculature may generate a number of gestational pathologies including miscarriages, intrauterine fetal death (IUFD), intrauterine growth restriction (IUGR), placental abruption, and preeclampsia. The importance of angiogenesis and angiogenetic factors in pregnancy is well known, and it has been proved that **chemokines and their receptors** are implicated in pregnancy and abortion, while cytokines and chemokines have a crucial part in controlling immune cells; these molecules are synthesized at the maternal-fetal interface where they have been implicated to play critical roles in the establishment and maintenance of pregnancy. In addition, they take part in other biological processes, such as cellular lymphoid organogenesis, and expression of adhesion molecules. The role of chemokines in angiogenesis during pregnancy has been experimentally demonstrated in cultures of leukocyte-free first trimester gestational decidual cells and in spontaneous miscarriage in mice, but the angiogenetic and angiostatic role of chemokines in the placental growth and decidua has not been well demonstrated [101–104]. These preliminary results propose a disturbance of the chemokine-associated angiogenetic network with a significant number of spontaneous abortions during the 1st trimester of gestation.

16. Conclusion

Miscarriage is the most usual complication of pregnancy. There are currently no definite predictive tests and treatments that can prevent spontaneous miscarriage. While 50% of miscarriages are associated with fetal chromosomal faults, most of the remaining cases are likely to be euploid fetuses that have failed due to implantation problems. Numerous investigators have previously figured that developing an accurate predictive test for miscarriage may open the window for identifying euploid pregnancies that are still viable but intended to miscarry. It follows therefore that possibly, emerging therapeutics could be targeted at such high risk euploid pregnancies so that some of them may continue to viability, (i.e., rescuing some from miscarriage). The treatment of miscarriages and especially RPL has a wide variety and should be targeted at the reason. It could be complicated to recommend general therapeutic management especially if they are unproven, invasive, and expensive, because most couples with unexplained recurrent miscarriages have a good outcome. Further investigation of the factors that regulate the possible transcriptional repression of angiogenic chemokines and/or the overexpression of the angiostatic chemokines could cooperate in early prediction and prevention of spontaneous abortions. We assume that an accurate investigation of chemokine networks possibly taking part in the angiogenetic mechanisms of pregnancy would assist in the design of more accurate and possibly individualized angiogenesis-associated strategies for improving the early prediction and prevention of spontaneous abortion.

Author details

Panagiotis Tsikouras[1*], Theodora Deftereou[1,3], Xanthoula Anthoulaki[1], Anastasia Bothou[1], Anna Chalkidou[1], Fotini Gaitatzi[1], Ioannis Tsirkas[1], Arsou Chalil Bourazan[1], Eirini Bampageorgaka[1], George Stanulov[1], Elefterios Chatzimichael[1], Spyridon Michalopoulos[1], Panagiotis Petsidis[2], Georgios Iatrakis[4], Stefanos Zervoudis[2], Maria Lambropoulou[3], Werner Rath[1,5] and Georgios Galazios[1]

1 Department of Obstetrics and Gynecology, Democritus University of Thrace, Greece

2 Department of Obstetrics and Gynecology, Rea Hospital, Athens, Greece

3 Department of Histology-Embryology, University Hospital Alexandroupolis, Greece

4 Department of Obstetrics and Gynecology, University of West Attica, Greece

5 Department of Obstetrics and Gynecology, University of Germany, Germany

*Address all correspondence to: ptsikour@med.duth.gr

References

[1] Brezina PR, Kutteh WH. Classic and cutting-edge strategies for the management of early pregnancy loss. Obstetrics and Gynecology Clinics of North America. 2014;**41**(1):1-18. DOI: 10.1016/j.ogc.2013.10.011. Epub: 12 December 2013

[2] Hatasaka HH. Recurrent miscarriage: Epidemiologic factors, definitions, and incidence. Clinical Obstetrics and Gynecology. 1994;**37**(3):625-634

[3] Hilden J, Modvig J, Damsgaard MT, Schmidt L. Estimation of the spontaneous abortion risk in the presence of induced abortions. Statistics in Medicine. 1991;**10**(2):285-297

[4] Modvig J, Schmidt L, Damsgaard MT. Measurement of total risk of spontaneous abortion: The virtue of conditional risk estimation. American Journal of Epidemiology. 1990;**132**(6):1021-1038

[5] Lathi RB, Gray Hazard FK, Heerema-McKenney A, Taylor J, Chueh JT. First trimester miscarriage evaluation. Seminars in Reproductive Medicine. 2011;**29**(6):463-469. DOI: 10.1055/s-0031-1293200. Epub: 8 December 2011

[6] Lund M, Kamper-Jørgensen M, Nielsen HS, Lidegaard Ø, Andersen AM, Christiansen OB. Prognosis for live birth in women with recurrent miscarriage: What is the best measure of success? Obstetrics and Gynecology. 2012;**119**(1):37-43. DOI: 10.1097/AOG.0b013e31823c0413

[7] Practice Committee of the American Society for Reproductive Medicine. Evaluation and treatment of recurrent pregnancy loss: A committee opinion. Fertility and Sterility. 2012;**98**(5):1103-1111. DOI: 10.1016/j.fertnstert.2012.06.048. Epub: 4 July 2012

[8] Stephenson MD. Frequency of factors associated with habitual abortion in 197 couples. Fertility and Sterility. 1996;**66**(1):24-29

[9] Practice Committee of the American Society for Reproductive Medicine. Aging and infertility in women. Fertility and Sterility. 2006;**86**(5 Suppl 1): S248-S252

[10] Nybo Andersen AM, Wohlfahrt J, Christens P, Olsen J, Melbye M. Maternal age and fetal loss: Population based register linkage study. British Medical Journal. 2000;**320**(7251):1708-1712

[11] Toth B, Würfel W, Bohlmann M, Zschocke J, Rudnik-Schöneborn S, Nawroth F, et al. Recurrent miscarriage: Diagnostic and therapeutic procedures. Guideline of the DGGG, OEGGG and SGGG (S2k-level, AWMF registry number 015/050). Geburtshilfe und Frauenheilkunde. 2018;**78**(4):364-381. DOI: 10.1055/a-0586-4568. Epub: 27 April 2018

[12] Toth B, Würfel W, Bohlmann MK, Gillessen-Kaesbach G, Nawroth F, Rogenhofer N, et al. Miscarriage: Diagnostic and therapeutic procedures. Guideline of the DGGG (S1-level, AWMF registry No. 015/050, December 2013). Geburtshilfe und Frauenheilkunde. 2015;**75**(11):1117-1129

[13] Preisler J, Kopeika J, Ismail L, Vathanan V, Farren J, Abdallah Y, et al. Defining safe criteria to diagnose miscarriage: Prospective observational multicentre study. British Medical Journal. 2015;**351**:h4579. DOI: 10.1136/bmj.h4579

[14] Bourne T, Bottomley C. When is a pregnancy nonviable and what criteria should be used to define miscarriage? Fertility and Sterility. 2012;**98**(5):1091-1096. DOI: 10.1016/j.fertnstert.2012.09.017

[15] Oates J, Casikar I, Campain A, Müller S, Yang J, Reid S, et al. A prediction model for viability at the end of the first trimester after a single early pregnancy evaluation. The Australian and New Zealand Journal of Obstetrics and Gynaecology. 2013;**53**(1):51-57. DOI: 10.1111/ajo.12046

[16] Pillai RN, Konje JC, Richardson M, Tincello DG, Potdar N. Prediction of miscarriage in women with viable intrauterine pregnancy—A systematic review and diagnostic accuracy meta-analysis. European Journal of Obstetrics, Gynecology, and Reproductive Biology. 2018;**220**:122-131. DOI: 10.1016/j.ejogrb.2017.10.024. Epub: 4 November 2017

[17] Christiansen OB. Research methodology in recurrent pregnancy loss. Obstetrics and Gynecology Clinics of North America. 2014;**41**(1):19-39. DOI: 10.1016/j.ogc.2013.10.001. Epub: 7 December 2013

[18] Choong S, Rombauts L, Ugoni A, Meagher S. Ultrasound prediction of risk of spontaneous miscarriage in live embryos from assisted conceptions. Ultrasound in Obstetrics and Gynecology. 2003;**22**(6):571-577

[19] Casikar I, Bignardi T, Riemke J, Alhamdan D, Condous G. Expectant management of spontaneous first-trimester miscarriage: Prospective validation of the '2-week rule'. Ultrasound in Obstetrics and Gynecology. 2010;**35**(2):223-227. DOI: 10.1002/uog.7486

[20] Stamatopoulos N, Lu C, Casikar I, Reid S, Mongelli M, Hardy N, et al. Prediction of subsequent miscarriage risk in women who present with a viable pregnancy at the first early pregnancy scan. The Australian and New Zealand Journal of Obstetrics and Gynaecology. 2015;**55**(5):464-472. DOI: 10.1111/ajo.12395. Epub : 21 August 2015

[21] Jauniaux E, Johns J, Burton GJ. The role of ultrasound imaging in diagnosing and investigating early pregnancy failure. Ultrasound in Obstetrics and Gynecology. 2005;**25**(6):613-624

[22] Sugiura-Ogasawara M, Ozaki Y, Katano K, Suzumori N, Mizutani E. Uterine anomaly and recurrent pregnancy loss. Seminars in Reproductive Medicine. 2011;**29**(6): 514-521. DOI: 10.1055/s-0031-1293205. Epub 2011 Dec 8

[23] Sugiura-Ogasawara M, Ozaki Y, Suzumori N. Müllerian anomalies and recurrent miscarriage. Current Opinion in Obstetrics and Gynecology. 2013;**25**(4):293-298. DOI: 10.1097/GCO.0b013e3283632849

[24] Sugiura-Ogasawara M, Ozaki Y, Kitaori T, Kumagai K, Suzuki S. Midline uterine defect size is correlated with miscarriage of euploid embryos in recurrent cases. Fertility and Sterility. 2010;**93**(6):1983-1988. DOI: 10.1016/j.fertnstert.2008.12.097. Epub: 27 February 2009

[25] Stovall DW, Parrish SB, Van Voorhis BJ, Hahn SJ, Sparks AE, Syrop CH. Uterine leiomyomas reduce the efficacy of assisted reproduction cycles: Results of a matched follow-up study. Human Reproduction. 1998;**13**(1):192-197

[26] Benecke C, Kruger TF, Siebert TI, Van der Merwe JP, Steyn DW. Effect of fibroids on fertility in patients undergoing assisted reproduction. A structured literature review. Gynecologic and Obstetric Investigation. 2005;**59**(4):225-230. Epub: 15 March 2005

[27] Jaslow CR, Kutteh WH. Effect of prior birth and miscarriage frequency on the prevalence of acquired and congenital uterine anomalies in women with recurrent miscarriage: A cross-sectional study. Fertility and Sterility.

2013;**99**(7):1916-22.e1. DOI: 10.1016/j.fertnstert.2013.01.152. Epub: 6 March 2013

[28] Jaslow CR. Uterine factors. Obstetrics and Gynecology Clinics of North America. 2014;**41**(1):57-86. DOI: 10.1016/j.ogc.2013.10.002

[29] Bailey AP, Jaslow CR, Kutteh WH. Minimally invasive surgical options for congenital and acquired uterine factors associated with recurrent pregnancy loss. Women's Health (London, England). 2015;**11**(2):161-167. DOI: 10.2217/whe.14.81

[30] Massalska D, Zimowski JG, Bijok J, Pawelec M, Czubak-Barlik M, Jakiel G, et al. First trimester pregnancy loss: Clinical implications of genetic testing. The Journal of Obstetrics and Gynaecology Research. 2017;**43**(1):23-29. DOI: 10.1111/jog.13179. Epub: 8 December 2016

[31] D'ippolito S, Di Simone N, Orteschi D, Pomponi MG, Genuardi M, Sisti LG, et al. The chromosome analysis of the miscarriage tissue. Miscarried embryo/fetal crown rump length (CRL) measurement: A practical use. PLoS ONE. 2017;**12**(6):e0178113. DOI: 10.1371/journal.pone.0178113. eCollection 2017

[32] Rubio C, Simón C, Vidal F, Rodrigo L, Pehlivan T, Remohí J, et al. Chromosomal abnormalities and embryo development in recurrent miscarriage couples. Human Reproduction. 2003;**18**(1):182-188

[33] Rubio C, Pehlivan T, Rodrigo L, Simón C, Remohí J, Pellicer A. Embryo aneuploidy screening for unexplained recurrent miscarriage: A minireview. American Journal of Reproductive Immunology. 2005;**53**(4):159-165

[34] Pagidas K, Ying Y, Keefe D. Predictive value of preimplantation genetic diagnosis for aneuploidy screening in repeated IVF-ET cycles among women with recurrent implantation failure. Journal of Assisted Reproduction and Genetics. 2008;**25**(2-3):103-106. DOI: 10.1007/s10815-008-9200-y. Epub: 12 February 2008

[35] Carp HJ, Dirnfeld M, Dor J, Grudzinskas JG. ART in recurrent miscarriage: Preimplantation genetic diagnosis/screening or surrogacy? Human Reproduction. 2004;**19**(7):1502-1505. Epub: 6 March 2004

[36] Brezina PR, Brezina DS, Kearns WG. Preimplantation genetic testing. British Medical Journal. 2012;**345**:e5908. DOI: 10.1136/bmj.e5908. Review

[37] Fragouli E, Wells D. Aneuploidy screening for embryo selection. Seminars in Reproductive Medicine. 2012;**30**(4):289-301. DOI: 10.1055/s-0032-1313908. Epub: 21 June 2012

[38] Andersen AM, Andersen PK, Olsen J, Grønbæk M, Strandberg-Larsen K. Moderate alcohol intake during pregnancy and risk of fetal death. International Journal of Epidemiology. 2012;**41**(2):405-413. DOI: 10.1093/ije/dyr189. Epub 2012 Jan 9

[39] Brent RL. Environmental causes of human congenital malformations: The pediatrician's role in dealing with these complex clinical problems caused by a multiplicity of environmental and genetic factors. Pediatrics. 2004;**113**(4 Suppl):957-968

[40] Ghazeeri GS, Kutteh WH. Autoimmune factors in reproductive failure. Current Opinion in Obstetrics and Gynecology. 2001;**13**(3):287-291

[41] Cervera R, Balasch J. Bidirectional effects on autoimmunity and reproduction. Human Reproduction Update. 2008;**14**(4):359-366. DOI: 10.1093/humupd/dmn013. Epub: 22 May 2008

[42] Kwak-Kim J, Agcaoili MS, Aleta L, Liao A, Ota K, Dambaeva S, et al. Management of women with recurrent pregnancy losses and antiphospholipid antibody syndrome. American Journal of Reproductive Immunology. 2013;**69**(6):596-607. DOI: 10.1111/aji.12114. Epub: 25 March 2013

[43] Schreiber K, Radin M, Sciascia S. Current insights in obstetric antiphospholipid syndrome. Current Opinion in Obstetrics and Gynecology. 2017;**29**(6):397-403. DOI: 10.1097/GCO.0000000000000406

[44] Arachchillage DR, Machin SJ, Mackie IJ, Cohen H. Diagnosis and management of non-criteria obstetric antiphospholipid syndrome. Thrombosis and Haemostasis. 2015;**113**(1):13-19. DOI: 10.1160/TH14-05-0416. Epub: 16 October 2014

[45] Han CS, Mulla MJ, Brosens JJ, Chamley LW, Paidas MJ, Lockwood CJ, et al. Aspirin and heparin effect on basal and antiphospholipid antibody modulation of trophoblast function. Obstetrics and Gynecology. 2011;**118**(5):1021-1028. DOI: 10.1097/AOG.0b013e31823234ad

[46] Quao ZC, Tong M, Bryce E, Guller S, Chamley LW, Abrahams VM. Low molecular weight heparin and aspirin exacerbate human endometrial endothelial cell responses to antiphospholipid antibodies. American Journal of Reproductive Immunology. 2018;**79**(1). DOI: 10.1111/aji.12785. Epub: 14 November 2017

[47] D'Ippolito S, Marana R, Di Nicuolo F, Castellani R, Veglia M, Stinson J, et al. PLoS ONE. 2012;**7**(1):e29660. DOI: 10.1371/journal.pone.0029660. Epub: 3 January 2012

[48] Tong S, Ngian GL, Onwude JL, Permezel M, Saglam B, Hay S, et al. Diagnostic accuracy of maternal serum macrophage inhibitory cytokine-1 and pregnancy-associated plasma protein—A at 6-10 weeks of gestation to predict miscarriage. Obstetrics and Gynecology. 2012;**119**(5):1000-1008. DOI: 10.1097/AOG.0b013e3182518fd3

[49] Huang C, Zhang H, Chen X, Diao L, Lian R, Zhang X, et al. Association of peripheral blood dendritic cells with recurrent pregnancy loss: A case-controlled study. American Journal of Reproductive Immunology. 2016;**76**(4):326-332. DOI: 10.1111/aji.12550. Epub: 21 August 2016

[50] Zhang C, Deng X, Zhang X, Pan Z, Zhao W, Zhang Y, et al. Association between serum TNF-α levels and recurrent spontaneous miscarriage: A meta-analysis. American Journal of Reproductive Immunology. 2016;**75**(2):86-93. DOI: 10.1111/aji.12447. Epub: 20 November 2015

[51] Smith ML, Schust DJ. Endocrinology and recurrent early pregnancy loss. Seminars in Reproductive Medicine. 2011;**29**(6):482-490. DOI: 10.1055/s-0031-1293202. Epub: 8 December 2011

[52] Krog MC, Nielsen HS, Christiansen OB, Kolte AM. Reproductive endocrinology in recurrent pregnancy loss. Clinical Obstetrics and Gynecology. 2016;**59**(3):474-486. DOI: 10.1097/GRF.0000000000000225

[53] Pluchino N, Drakopoulos P, Wenger JM, Petignat P, Streuli I, Genazzani AR. Hormonal causes of recurrent pregnancy loss (RPL). Hormones (Athens, Greece). 2014;**13**(3):314-322. DOI: 10.14310/horm.2002.1505

[54] Dean DD, Agarwal S, Tripathi P. Connecting links between genetic factors defining ovarian reserve and recurrent miscarriages. Journal of Assisted Reproduction and Genetics. 2018;**35**(12):2121-2128. DOI: 10.1007/s10815-018-1305-3. Epub: 15 September 2018

[55] Alexander EK, Pearce EN, Brent GA, Brown RS, Chen H, Dosiou C. 2017 guidelines of the American Thyroid Association for the diagnosis and management of thyroid disease during pregnancy and the postpartum. Thyroid. 2017;**27**(3):315-389. DOI: 10.1089/thy.2016.0457

[56] Greene MF. Spontaneous abortions and major malformations in women with diabetes mellitus. Seminars in Reproductive Endocrinology. 1999;**17**(2):127-136

[57] Dlugi AM. Hyperprolactinemic recurrent spontaneous pregnancy loss: A true clinical entity or a spurious finding? Fertility and Sterility. 1998;**70**(2):253-255

[58] Coulam CB, Acacio B. Does immunotherapy for treatment of reproductive failure enhance live births? American Journal of Reproductive Immunology. 2012;**67**(4):296-304. DOI: 10.1111/j.1600-0897.2012.01111.x. Epub: 16 February 2012

[59] Younis JS. Ovarian aging and implications for fertility female health. Minerva Endocrinologica. 2012;**37**(1):41-57

[60] Ke RW. Endocrine basis for recurrent pregnancy loss. Obstetrics and Gynecology Clinics of North America. 2014;**41**(1):103-112. DOI: 10.1016/j.ogc.2013.10.003. Epub: 5 December 2013

[61] Jauniaux E, Farquharson RG, Christiansen OB, Exalto N. Evidence-based guidelines for the investigation and medical treatment of recurrent miscarriage. Human Reproduction. 2006;**21**(9):2216-2222. Epub: 17 May 2006

[62] van Wely M, Bayram N, van der Veen F, Bossuyt PM. Predictors for treatment failure after laparoscopic electrocautery of the ovaries in women with clomiphene citrate resistant polycystic ovary syndrome. Human Reproduction. 2005;**20**(4):900-905. Epub: 7 January 2005

[63] Nahuis MJ, Kose N, Bayram N, van Dessel HJ, Braat DD, Hamilton CJ, et al. Long-term outcomes in women with polycystic ovary syndrome initially randomized to receive laparoscopic electrocautery of the ovaries or ovulation induction with gonadotrophins. Human Reproduction. 2011;**26**(7):1899-1904. DOI: 10.1093/humrep/der141. Epub: 15 May 2011

[64] Morley LC, Tang T, Yasmin E, Norman RJ, Balen AH. Polycystic ovary syndrome, the G1691A factor V Leiden mutation, and plasminogen activator inhibitor activity: Associations with recurrent pregnancy loss. Cochrane Database of Systematic Reviews. 2017;**11**:CD003053. DOI: 10.1002/14651858.CD003053.pub6.

[65] Glueck CJ, Wang P, Bornovali S, Goldenberg N, Sieve L. Insulin-sensitising drugs (metformin, rosiglitazone, pioglitazone, D-chiro-inositol) for women with polycystic ovary syndrome, oligo amenorrhoea and subfertility. Metabolism. 2003;**52**(12):1627-1632

[66] Legro RS, Barnhart HX, Schlaff WD, Carr BR, Diamond MP, Carson SA, et al. Cooperative multicenter reproductive medicine network. Clomiphene, metformin, or both for infertility in the polycystic ovary syndrome. The New England Journal of Medicine. 2007;**356**(6):551-566

[67] Jovanovic L, Knopp RH, Kim H, Cefalu WT, Zhu XD, Lee YJ, et al. Elevated pregnancy losses at high and low extremes of maternal glucose in early normal and diabetic pregnancy: Evidence for a protective adaptation in diabetes. Diabetes Care. 2005;**28**(5):1113-1117

[68] Ben Ayed B, Dammak dit Mlik S, Ben Arab H, Trabelssi H, Chahtour H,

Mathlouthi N, et al. Metformin effects on clomifene-induced ovulation in the polycystic ovary syndrome. Journal Medical Tunisie. 2009;**87**(1):43-49

[69] Hay PE. Bacterial vaginosis and miscarriage. Current Opinion in Infectious Diseases. 2004;**17**(1):41-44

[70] Donders GG, Van Calsteren K, Bellen G, Reybrouck R, Van den Bosch T, et al. Predictive value for preterm birth of abnormal vaginal flora, bacterial vaginosis and aerobic vaginitis during the first trimester of pregnancy. BJOG: An International Journal of Obstetrics and Gynaecology. 2009;**116**(10):1315-1324. DOI: 10.1111/j.1471-0528.2009.02237.x. Epub: 17 June 2009

[71] Vrbanac A, Riestra AM, Coady A, Knight R, Nizet V, Patras KA. The murine vaginal microbiota and its perturbation by the human pathogen group B streptococcus. BMC Microbiology. 2018;**18**(1):197. DOI: 10.1186/s12866-018-1341-2

[72] Purwar M, Ughade S, Bhagat B, Agarwal V, Kulkarni H. Bacterial vaginosis in early pregnancy and adverse pregnancy outcome. The Journal of Obstetrics and Gynaecology Research. 2001;**27**(4):175-181

[73] McDonald HM, Brocklehurst P, Gordon A. Antibiotics for treating bacterial vaginosis in pregnancy. Cochrane Database of Systematic Reviews. 2013;(1):CD000262

[74] Workowski KA, Bolan GA. Centers for disease control and prevention. Sexually transmitted diseases treatment guidelines, 2015. MMWR—Recommendations and Reports. 2015;**64**(RR-03):1-137

[75] Saravelos SH, Li TC. Unexplained recurrent miscarriage: How can we explain it? Human Reproduction. 2012;**27**(7):1882-1886. DOI: 10.1093/humrep/des102. Epub: 2 May 2012

[76] Kaandorp SP, van Mens TE, Middeldorp S, Hutten BA, Hof MH, van der Post JA, et al. Time to conception and time to live birth in women with unexplained recurrent miscarriage. Human Reproduction. 2014;**29**(6):1146-1152. DOI: 10.1093/humrep/deu052. Epub: 28 March 2014

[77] Pillai RN, Konje JC, Tincello DG, Potdar N. Role of serum biomarkers in the prediction of outcome in women with threatened miscarriage: A systematic review and diagnostic accuracy meta-analysis. Human Reproduction Update. 2016;**22**(2):228-239. DOI: 10.1093/humupd/dmv054. Epub: 9 December 2015

[78] Davenport WB, Kutteh WH. Inherited thrombophilias and adverse pregnancy outcomes: A review of screening patterns and recommendations. Obstetrics and Gynecology Clinics of North America. 2014;**41**(1):133-144. DOI: 10.1016/j.ogc.2013.10.005. Epub: 10 December 2013

[79] American College of Obstetricians and Gynecologists Women's Health Care Physicians. ACOG practice bulletin No. 138: Inherited thrombophilias in pregnancy. Obstetrics and Gynecology. 2013;**122**(3):706-717. DOI: 10.1097/01.AOG.0000433981.36184.4e

[80] Battinelli EM, Bauer KA. Thrombophilias in pregnancy. Hematology/Oncology Clinics of North America. 2011;**25**(2):323-333. DOI: 10.1016/j.hoc.2011.02.003

[81] Said JM, Higgins JR, Moses EK, Walker SP, Monagle PT, Brennecke SP. Inherited thrombophilias and adverse pregnancy outcomes: A case-control study in an Australian population. Acta Obstetricia et Gynecologica Scandinavica. 2012;**91**(2):250-255. DOI: 10.1111/j.1600-0412.2011.01293.x. Epub: 9 November 2011

[82] Rodger MA, Walker MC, Smith GN, Wells PS, Ramsay T, Langlois NJ, et al. Is thrombophilia associated with placenta-mediated pregnancy complications? A prospective cohort study. Journal of Thrombosis and Haemostasis. 2014;**12**(4):469-478. DOI: 10.1111/jth.12509

[83] Kutteh WH, Triplett DA. Thrombophilias and recurrent pregnancy loss. Seminars in Reproductive Medicine. 2006;**24**(1):54-66

[84] Luxembourg B, Lindhoff-Last E. Genomic diagnosis of thrombophilia in women: Clinical relevance. Hämostaseologie. 2007;**27**(1):22-31

[85] Kupferminc MJ, Eldor A, Steinman N, Many A, Bar-Am A, Jaffa A, et al. Increased frequency of genetic thrombophilia in women with complications of pregnancy. The New England Journal of Medicine. 1999;**340**(1):9-13

[86] James A. Committee on practice bulletins—Obstetrics. Practice bulletin no. 123: Thromboembolism in pregnancy. Obstetrics and Gynecology. 2011;**118**(3):718-729. DOI: 10.1097/AOG.0b013e3182310c4c

[87] Martí-Carvajal AJ, Solà I, Lathyris D, Dayer M. Homocysteine-lowering interventions for preventing cardiovascular events. Cochrane Database of Systematic Reviews. 2017;**8**:CD006612. DOI: 10.1002/14651858.CD006612.pub5

[88] Stanger O, Herrmann W, Pietrzik K, Fowler B, Geisel J, Dierkes J, et al. Clinical use and rational management of homocysteine, folic acid, and B vitamins in cardiovascular and thrombotic diseases. Zeitschrift für Kardiologie. 2004;**93**(6):439-453

[89] Rugolo S, Mirabella D, Cantone SM, Giuffrida A. Hyperhomocysteinemia: Associated obstetric diabetes and fetal malformations. Minerva Ginecologica. 2005;**57**(6):619-625

[90] Aubard Y, Darodes N, Cantaloube M. Hyperhomocysteinemia and pregnancy—Review of our present understanding and therapeutic implications. European Journal of Obstetrics, Gynecology, and Reproductive Biology. 2000;**93**(2):157-165

[91] Taylor BV, Oudit GY, Evans M. Homocysteine, vitamins, and coronary artery disease. Comprehensive review of the literature. Canadian Family Physician. 2000;**46**:2236-2245

[92] Diaz-Hernandez JI, Moncada S, Bolaños JP, Almeida A. Poly(ADP-ribose) polymerase-1 protects neurons against apoptosis induced by oxidative stress. Cell Death and Differentiation. 2007;**14**(6):1211-1221. Epub: 9 March 2007

[93] Czeizel AE. Periconceptional folic acid and multivitamin supplementation for the prevention of neural tube defects and other congenital abnormalities. Birth Defects Research. Part A, Clinical and Molecular Teratology. 2009;**85**(4):260-268. DOI: 10.1002/bdra.20563

[94] Coumans AB, Huijgens PC, Jakobs C, Schats R, de Vries JI, van Pampus MG, et al. Haemostatic and metabolic abnormalities in women with unexplained recurrent abortion. Human Reproduction. 1999;**14**(1):211-214

[95] Facchinetti F, Marozio L, Frusca T, Grandone E, Venturini P, Tiscia GL, et al. Maternal thrombophilia and the risk of recurrence of preeclampsia. American Journal of Obstetrics and Gynecology. 2009;**200**(1):46.e1-46.e5. DOI: 10.1016/j.ajog.2008.07.032. Epub: 9 October 2008

[96] Powers RW, Evans RW, Ness RB, Crombleholme WR, Roberts JM. Homocysteine and cellular fibronectin are increased in preeclampsia, not transient hypertension

of pregnancy. Hypertension in Pregnancy. 2001;**20**(1):69-77

[97] Powers RW, Evans RW, Majors AK, Ojimba JI, Ness RB, Crombleholme WR, et al. Plasma homocysteine concentration is increased in preeclampsia and is associated with evidence of endothelial activation. American Journal of Obstetrics and Gynecology. 1998;**179**(6 Pt 1):1605-1611

[98] Ray JG, Laskin CA. Folic acid and homocyst(e)ine metabolic defects and the risk of placental abruption, pre-eclampsia and spontaneous pregnancy loss: A systematic review. Placenta. 1999;**20**(7):519-529

[99] Mtiraoui N, Zammiti W, Ghazouani L, Braham NJ, Saidi S, Finan RR, et al. Methylenetetrahydrofolate reductase C677T and A1298C polymorphism and changes in homocysteine concentrations in women with idiopathic recurrent pregnancy losses. Reproduction. 2006;**131**(2):395-401

[100] Wiwanitkit V. Roles of methylenetetrahydrofolate reductase C677T polymorphism in repeated pregnancy loss. Clinical and Applied Thrombosis/Hemostasis. 2005;**11**(3):343-345

[101] Musters AM, Koot YE, van den Boogaard NM, Kaaijk E, Macklon NS, van der Veen F, et al. Supportive care for women with recurrent miscarriage: A survey to quantify women's preferences. Human Reproduction. 2013;**28**(2):398-405. DOI: 10.1093/humrep/des374. Epub: 4 December 2012

[102] van den Berg MMJ, Dancet EAF, Erlikh T, van der Veen F, Goddijn M, Hajenius PJ. Patient-centered early pregnancy care: A systematic review of quantitative and qualitative studies on the perspectives of women and their partners. Human Reproduction Update. 2018;**24**(1):106-118. DOI: 10.1093/humupd/dmx030

[103] Van den Berg MM, Vissenberg R, Goddijn M. Recurrent miscarriage clinics. Obstetrics and Gynecology Clinics of North America. 2014 Mar;**41**(1):145-155. DOI: 10.1016/j.ogc.2013.10.010. Epub: 15 December 2013

[104] Van Den Boogaard E, Hermens RP, Leschot NJ, Baron R, Vollebergh JH, Bernardus RE, et al. Identification of barriers for good adherence to a guideline on recurrent miscarriage. Acta Obstetricia et Gynecologica Scandinavica. 2011;**90**(2):186-191. DOI: 10.1111/j.1600-0412.2010.01000.x. Epub: 2 December 2010

Chapter 6

Interruption of Pregnancy in Women with the Uterine Scar: Potential Risks

Galina Dikke and Vladimir Ostromenskiy

Abstract

Summary objective: To assess the risks and identify effective and safe methods of abortion in women with uterine scar. Material: Literary sources published in the databases of Medline, PubMed, and others, of which 57 are included in this review. The main provisions: Termination of pregnancy in women with a scar on the uterus involves the use of any available method. For women with a scar on the uterus, it is necessary to prepare the cervix before a surgical abortion in all terms. Abnormal implantation of the embryo within the fibrous tissue of the scar after caesarean section can cause life-threatening bleeding of the mother during or after the termination of the pregnancy. Surgical excision of the affected area by hysteroscopic access, as well as transvaginal or transabdominal local administration of Methotrexate with or without an additional intramuscular dose of the same drug, seems to be optimal from the point of view of minimizing the frequency of complications. Conclusion: A scar on the uterus after caesarean section presents a high risk of abnormal attachment of the ovum and fatal bleeding during abortion.

Keywords: medical abortion, surgical abortion, uterine scar, bleeding

1. Introduction

Interruption of pregnancy in patients with uterine scar, as well as in women without it, can be artificial (in early and late pregnancy period if medically required, and also in pregnancy period exceeding 22 weeks—at still birth) or spontaneous.

Although there is no doubt presently that now caesarean section is quite a safe procedure, it still presents a certain risk not only for the subsequent pregnancy and confinement, but also in case of its interruption.

Interruption of pregnancy in women with uterine scar assumes the use of any accessible method [1]. However, the abortion made by the method of uterine curettage in the interval period aggravates the forecast. The risk of scar inadequacy in this case increases 1.5 times.

Recently, substantial growth of registered cases of localisation of ovum in the uterine scar after previous caesarean section has been observed [2]. After one or several caesarean section operations, the specific localisation of the chorion, such as presentation and scar increta, can be a reason of serious complications during and after interruption of pregnancy.

2. Medicamentous interruption of pregnancy in women with an uterine scar

The technology of medicamentous interruption of pregnancy in the early period, the used preparations and their doses do not differ for groups of women having a uterine scar and those without it.

It is marked in medical periodicals that the use of Mifepristone and Misoprostol for interruption of pregnancy during the period not later than 49 days of amenorrhoea in women with a uterine scar is safe and effective [3, 4]. Not a single case of uterine rupture at the place of the scar or increased frequency of other complications is described for medicamentous interruption of pregnancy in early period in case of caesarean section in the anamnesis, in comparison with the women who did not undergo operative uterine treatment [5].

The preceding caesarean section operations are deemed to be a uterine rupture risk factor in case of interrupting gestation at 13 weeks and later. However, the study of abortion results in the second trimester, induced by Misoprostol, in 720 women with one or several prior caesarean section intervention shows that the use of the medicamentous method does not cause more frequent complications in comparison with the women with non-operated uterine (the absolute risk of uterine rupture is $<0.4\%$) [1].

Thus, the presence of a uterine scar after the previous caesarean section is not a contraindication for medical abortion at early pregnancy and does not involve increased frequency of complications.

3. Recommendations for medical abortion in women after caesarean section in case of localisation of the chorion/placenta outside the uterine scar

- The most essential data for medicamentous interruption of pregnancy relate to the application of Misoprostol, but the level of evidence is low. The doses of Misoprostol in case of late pregnancy interruption should be twice lower for the women with uterine scar, in comparison with the women without it (**Table 1**) [6].

- The use of Mifepristone or hygroscopic dilators is not counter-indicative [7].

- In case of interruption of late pregnancy or foetus death in patients with the uterine scar, in most cases induction of confinement is more preferable than planned caesarean section irrespective of the number of past caesarean section operations (the recommendation of a professional consensus).

- In case of still birth, at the period of 27–28 and over 28 weeks of gestation, Misoprostol is not used for medicamentous abortion [6].

- The presently practiced options of medical treatment of women with incomplete or missed abortion include expectant management (for women with spontaneous miscarriage, with no excessive uterine bleeding, with stable haemodynamics and no signs of infection), medicamentous treatment (usually Misoprostol or Mifepristone/Misoprostol) or surgical treatment (vacuum aspiration or dilation and curettage). An important factor in choosing a method for management of spontaneous miscarriage is the woman's preference [8, 9].

- In case of non-developing pregnancy up to 63 days of amenorrhoea, only the use of Misoprostol at a dose of 800 mcg vaginally or 600 mcg sublingually is possible. Administration can be repeated in 3 hours, if necessary (2 doses maximum).

- The patients with a uterine scar willing to interrupt the pregnancy or those with unexpected miscarriage, need all-round detailed consultation, and the doctor must consider all variants of administration, their advantages and risks. Individual approach is necessary, with account of the obstetric anamnesis, comorbid diseases and potential complications, such as haemorrhage and uterine rupture constituting a life-threatening situation [1].

Advanced pregnancy, no previous confinement in the past medical history and previous confinement by caesarean section result in extended duration of abortion.

The mother's age, body mass index, race and the interval between administration of Mifepristone and Misoprostol do not affect the duration of the abortion.

Preparation of the cervix before surgical abortion is recommended to all women with the pregnancy exceeding 12–14 weeks. The preparation can be recommended as well to women with high risk of cervix trauma or uterine perforation at any pregnancy period. For this purpose, osmotic dilators (laminaria tents, Dilapan-S), pharmacological medications (Mifepristone, Misoprostol) or their combinations are used.

Preparation	Dose	Method of administration	Frequency of administration
Up to 49 days*	400 μg	Orally	One time
50–63 days*	800 μg	Vaginally***	One time
64–84 days*	800 μg 400 μg	Vaginally*** (first dose), subsequently vaginally*** or sublingually	Every 3 hours, up to 4 doses
If abortion fails to occur within 14 days, then vacuum aspiration is administered			
13–24 weeks*	200 μg	Vaginally*** (first dose), sublingually (subsequent doses)	Every 3 hours, up to interruption of pregnancy
If abortion fails to occur within 24 hours, then administration of Mifepristone is to be repeated in 3 hours after the last dose of Misoprostol, and after 12 hours-Misoprostol			
25–26 weeks*	100 μg	Vaginally,*** buccally or sublingually	Every 4 hours (in case of still birth-after 6 hours), up to interruption of pregnancy
An extra dose Misoprostol is applied if the placenta did not come off in 30 minutes after foetus expulsion			
27–28 weeks**	100 μg	Vaginally,*** buccally or sublingually	Every 4 hours, up to interruption of pregnancy
Over 28 weeks**	50 μg	Vaginally,*** buccally or sublingually	Every 6 hours, up to interruption of pregnancy
An extra dose Misoprostol is applied if the placenta did not come off in 30 minutes after foetus expulsion			

Misoprostol is applied in 24–48 hours after administration of Mifepristone at a dose 200 mg one time ingestion.
**Is not applied in case of still birth.*
***To exclude vaginal application in case of haemorrhage or signs of infection.*

Table 1.
Medical abortion schemes with application of misoprostol in women with a uterine scar [6].

The advantages of osmotic dilators over Mifepristone or Misoprostol have been identified in terms of efficiency [10–12], of Dilapan-S over laminaria tents in the accepted "one-day" procedures for cervical dilatation [13] and in respect of the use of Misoprostol in addition to osmotic dilators in case of cervix deformation or pregnancy period exceeding 16 weeks [14].

In some cases, osmotic dilators are used more extensively, for instance, in treatment of teenagers, non-parous women or women with cervical scars. It is also recommended to increase the number of dilators with the progress of pregnancy period. As compared with laminaria tents, by-half-less number of Dilapan-S rods is required because of wider cervical dilatation [14]. Two rods are recommended at the 13–15-week pregnancy period, three at 16–18-week period and four at 18 weeks-period and further (though only few proofs substantiate this recommendation). After 18 weeks, administration of Dilapan-S is recommended one time overnight [15]. However, one rod inserted 3–4 hours prior to the dilation and evacuation can be sufficient for the pregnancy period not exceeding 18 weeks.

The methods combining osmotic dilators and Misoprostol are efficient owing to the shortest known time to yield effect (from 2 to 4 hours). The possibility to complete the procedure within 1 day for the 18–22 weeks pregnancy period was demonstrated by Lyus R. et al., who used 3 Dilapan-S rods and 400 μg of Misoprostol. The average time for preparation of the cervix was 3 hours 40 minutes, and the average time of the manipulation—10 minutes [16].

The preparation of the cervix at the 17–22 weeks period of pregnancy requires greater time, sometimes 2–3 days (with replacement of dilators) [17]. The comparison of Dilapan-S with laminaria tents showed that the adequate cervical dilation on the 2nd day was achieved in 98 and 56% of women respectively [18].

4. Chorion ingrowth into the uterine scar in early pregnancy

Accreta, increta and percreta of the chorion is characterized by their accretion to the uterine myometrium without any intermediate decidual membrane, with different extent of their invasion into the myometrium. In the scientific literature, the term "placenta accreta" incorporates "placenta increta et percreta".

4.1 Epidemiology

The chorion ingrowth into the uterine scar during the early pregnancy is diagnosed extremely seldom and varies between 1/110 and 1/2500 of pregnancy cases [19]. Some authors note a gradual increase in placentation anomalies, which coincides in proportion with the increased frequency of caesarean section operations: in 1970s years the figure was 1/70,000 [20], and in 2005—1/533 [21]. The meta-analysis made for the period from 1972 to 2011 describes 47 cases of diagnosed placentation anomalies in the first trimester and at the beginning of the second trimester [22].

4.2 Complications of artificial abortion in case of chorion increta into the uterine scar

According to Abbas et al. [23], placenta accreta is usually not identified in the first trimester of pregnancy, and the diagnosis concerning this pathology is made retrospectively for patients with excessive haemorrhage that arises during the uterine curettage which is secondary in relation to the invasion of chorionic villi in the myometrium [23]. Some observations of tardive uterine bleeding in some weeks and even several years after the abortion [24, 25] have been described.

According to Jang et al., the clinical manifestation may also include spontaneous uterine rupture with clinical development of "sharp belly" and haemoperitoneum [26]. Spontaneous uterine rupture was registered in 15 out of 47 cases (32%) described in the meta-analysis; most of them were asymptomatic and were accompanied by intra-abdominal haemorrhage and collapse [22].

The form of abnormal embryo implantation in the scar fibrous tissue after the caesarean section, dangerous for the mother's life, can lead to ectopic pregnancy (localisation of the ovum between the uterus and it serous membrane). The diagnostics of such condition with the help of ultrasonography does not represent any difficulties and is made for pregnancy period of 5–12 weeks, with the time interval between the last caesarean section and the ectopic pregnancy from 6 months to 12 years [27].

The complications associated with chorion increta also include fistulisation, infection, perinatal and maternal death [28].

4.3 Diagnostics of chorion increta into the uterine scar in early pregnancy

The review of literature devoted to the issue of early diagnostics of chorion ingrowth into the uterine scar, made by Timor-Tritsch et al. [22], showed that this diagnostics is quite complicated. The other authors also note that placental accreta, increta or percreta in the first trimester of pregnancy is identified with difficultly [4, 24]. The literature refers only to several cases of diagnosed placenta accreta in the first trimester of pregnancy [23].

Most publications include information on placentation anomalies in the first trimester diagnosed during the morphological examination of the uterus ablated because of excessive bleeding that took place during the uterine curettage in early pregnancy or within a tardive period after the abortion.

No objective signs of chorion increta into the uterine scar are present.

Chorion increta risk factors (*present in past medical history*): uterine scar (caesarean section or myomectomy), manual ectomy of placenta, multiple gestation, dilation and curettage, endometriosis, multiple confinement, advanced age of the mother, IVF induced pregnancy.

The actual dependence of the chorion/placenta increta frequency on the specified risk factors remains obscure. The combination of two-three and more factors is observed for most cases of placenta percreta [29]. In case of placenta presentation to the scar, the ingrowth risk makes 3% after the first caesarean section and reaches 40% and more after the third similar operation [30].

4.3.1 Ultrasonography

Diagnostics of ovum localisation in the uterine cavity, as viewed by ultrasonography, is an integral part of diagnosing uterine pregnancy and usually does not present any complexity.

Sonography is a very important instrument for exact location of the gestational sac and for diagnosing inadequacy of the postoperative uterine scar.

The ultrasonic signs of chorion ingrowth into the uterine scar in the first trimester are as follows (**Figures 1–4**):

- absence of decidual membrane in the area of localisation of the placenta
- low-lying gestational sac (in the scar area)
- invagination of the placenta towards the bladder

- hypoechoic inclusions (lacunae) in the placental area
- myometrium thickness in the retroplacental zone below 1 mm
- more intense uterine-placental blood flow.

Sensibility—41%, specificity—88% [19]. For comparison: these indices in the second trimester make 60 and 83.5% respectively.

Histopathologically, chorion increta (irrespective of having a uterine scar) is characterized by partial or complete **absence of decidual membrane**, following which the placental villi get accreted to the myometrium or invade it (**Figure 1**).

According to Richardson et al. [31], the "key" to identifying chorion increta lies in the retroplacental complex and is characterized by **absence of a hypoechogenic line** (**the norm being from 1 to 2 mm**), that is, there is a loss of normal decidual interaction between the chorion and the myometrium (**Figure 2**).

The presence of placental lacunae (**Figures 3** and **4**), according to some authors, is the most valuable attribute of placenta increta, with the 89% sensibility, specificity of 81%, positive prognostic value of 73% and negative prognostic value of 93% [32], while the combination of lacunae and myometrium thickness below 1 mm in the retroplacental complex zone shows the metrics of 100, 72, 72 and 100% respectively [33].

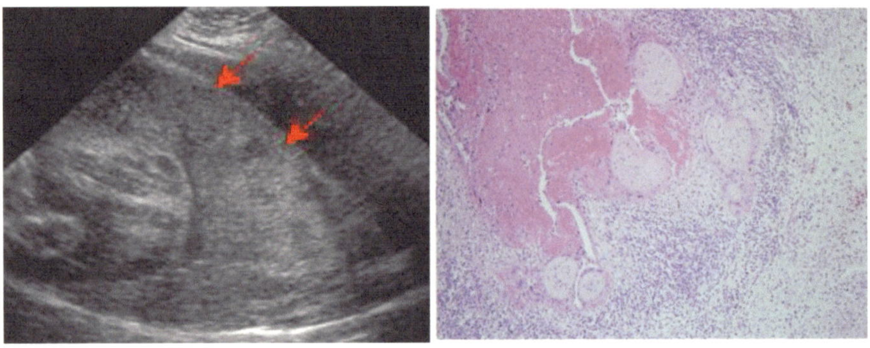

Figure 1.
On the left: ultrasonographic examination-absence of decidual membrane in the placental localisation area; on the right: histopathological examination—chorionic villi in the myometrium with no decidual membrane (haematoxylin, eosin; 100×) [24].

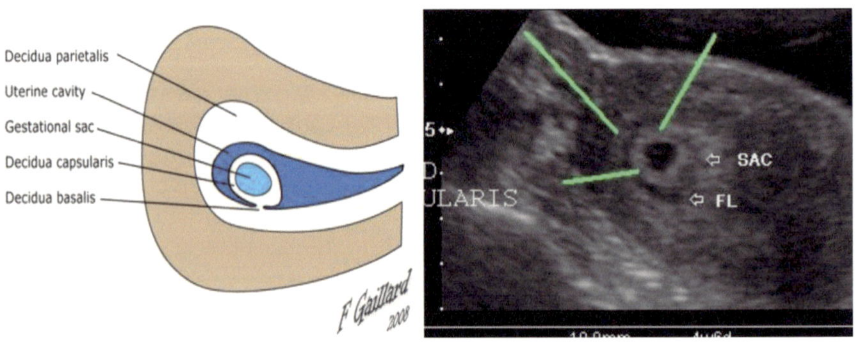

Figure 2.
Ultrasonographic examination: retroplacental complex (on the left: the scheme; on the right: designated with arrows from the left to the right—decidua capsularis, decidua parietalis, decidua basalis; other denotations: SAC—gestational sac, FL—fluid-containing space—hypoechogenic line between decidua parietalis and decidua basalis).

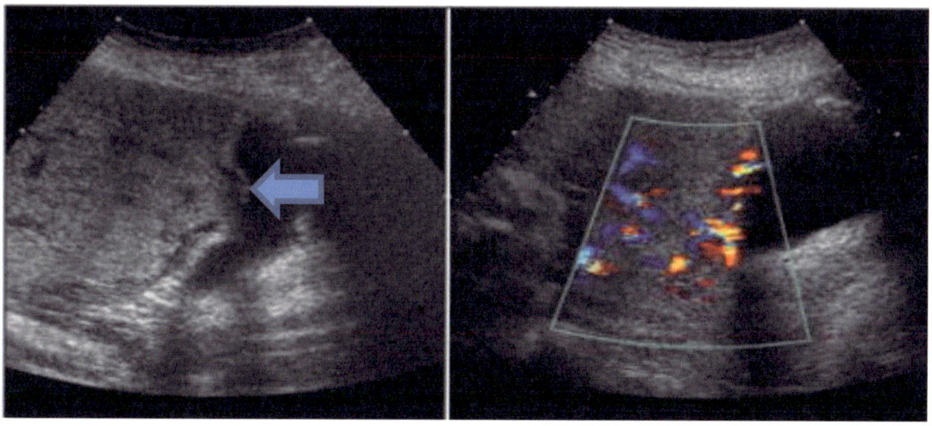

Figure 3.
Ultrasonographic examination: on the left—sonogram, grey scale: evagination of the placenta into the bladder; on the right—sonogram, colour doppler: visible hypervascularisation between the uterine serous membrane and the bladder wall; placental lacunae [34].

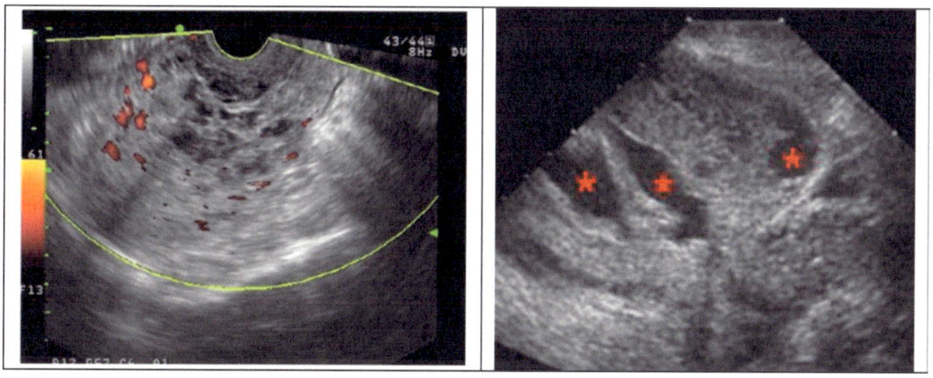

Figure 4.
Ultrasonographic examination: hypoechoic inclusions (lacunae) in the placental area (composite cystophorous "aggregate" in the uterine wall) [34].

The uterine scar inadequacy is diagnosed not only and not purely on the basis of thinning of the scar and the presence of considerable number of hyperechoic inclusions (connective tissue), but also by exposure **of other ultrasonic markers** which include: visualisation of total defect of the myometrium in the scar projection, in the form of a "niche" from the uterine cavity side, reaching the serous membrane; or partial defect in the myometrium in the scar projection, in the form of a "niche", with thinning of the lower uterine segment down to 3 mm and below; myometrium deformation with retraction from the uterine serous membrane side and a "niche" from the uterine cavity side, with thinning of the unchanged myometrium down to 3 mm and below; total, subtotal necrosis of the myometrium. The enumerated criteria are deemed to be an indication for operative treatment of the inadequate uterine scar during the period of periconceptional preparation.

The value of uterine scar thickness indicator or other criteria of inadequacy as predictors of uterine rupture and excessive bleeding in the first trimester of pregnancy in case of its interruption, has not been studied and is not known. Most of the echographic criteria of placenta increta have a real diagnostic value only after 15 weeks of pregnancy (sensibility—78–93%, after 28 weeks—100%).

In the absence of a clear picture or in case of doubtful ultrasonographic results at suspicion on ectopic pregnancy, other methods of research are undertaken.

4.3.2 Magnetic resonance imaging

To diagnose placenta increta in the second and third trimesters of pregnancy, magnetic resonance imaging (MRI) is used in recent years in case of dubious results of ultrasonography [22]. However, diagnostics with the help of ultrasonography (including colour Doppler) and MRI has not shown a statistically significant difference [35]. No valid criteria of MRI diagnostics are so far developed.

An observation of a 41-year-old patient with a caesarean section in the past medical history has been described. The patient had an intra-abdominal haemorrhage on the 21st week of pregnancy, without any signs of placental anomalies according to the ultrasonography data, whereas the MRI showed a picture of deep placental invasion suggesting placenta increta or percreta (**Figure 5**). Placenta percreta was confirmed by the histological examination of the operatively extirpated uterus (ablated in connection with spontaneous uterine rupture during the confinement) [28].

An observation of a 42-year-old patient with vaginal haemorrhage and pain in the lower abdomen lasting for 2 weeks after the dilation and curettage, at the 5-week gestation period, has been described. The level of β-HCG in serum was 2009.3 mlU/ml. The diagnosis—chorionic increta—was made on the basis of magnetic resonance imaging (**Figure 6**).

The sensibility of magnetic resonance imaging is 77%, the specificity—50% in patients with average 30.8 weeks period of pregnancy. The accuracy of diagnosis makes 67% [36]. As to the earlier gestation periods, no data were found for the specified parameters.

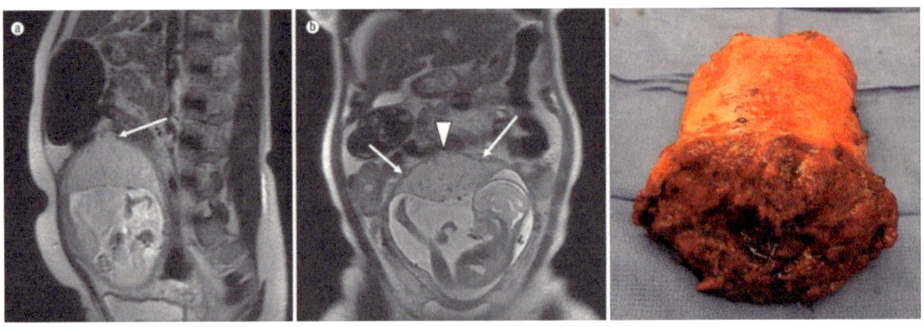

Figure 5.
Patient N. aged 41. Magnetic resonance imaging (on the left): (a) sagittal MR image-deep placental invasion (the arrow); (b) coronal MR image of placenta (the arrowhead), invasion extending deep into the surrounding myometrium (the arrows). Gross specimen (on the right): extirpated uterus [28].

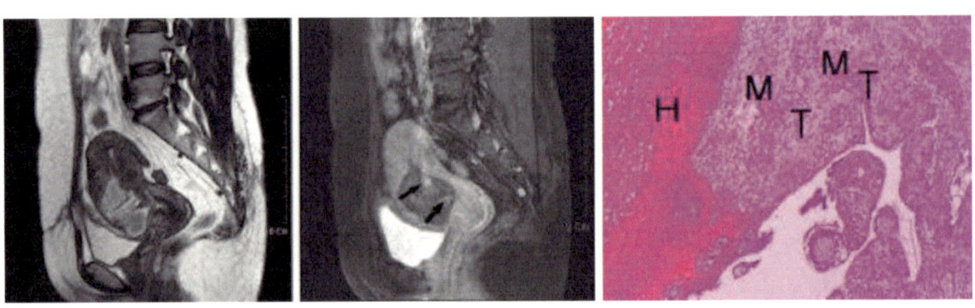

Figure 6.
Patient R., 42 years old. Magnetic resonance imaging (on the left): A-sagittal T2-weighted MR image (TR/TE 4000/85 ms) of the pelvic area shows a clearly contoured intramyometric aggregate with high signal intensity. B-sagittal T1-weighted MR image (TR/TE 150/4.2 ms)—after intravenous administration of gadolinium-based contrast medium, shows a hypointense aggregate with focal areas of intensification (the arrows). Morphological examination (on the right): Invasion of trophoblast (T) in the myometrium (M), accompanied by a haematoma (H) [37].

5. Management of patients with ingrowth of chorion into the uterine scar in case of interrupting pregnancy in early periods

The scientific literature describes a clinical observation [38] of a woman with two caesarean section operations in the past history. The reviewed pregnancy was third, 11th week. The patient entered the hospital with excessive uterine haemorrhage. The nonsurgical arrangements (uterine curettage, etc.) proved to be inefficient, therefore she was subjected to hysterectomy. The total blood loss was estimated to be 3500–4000 ml. The haemoglobin figure was 8.1 g/dl. Transfusion of 9 units of erythrocytes and 4 units of fresh frozen plasma was effected. The patient recovered from the critical condition and was discharged on 7th day after the operation. The histopathological examination of the specimen (the extirpated uterus) confirmed the diagnosis "placenta accreta".

Takeda et al. [25] describe a clinical observation of placenta increta in a 27-year-old woman (three pregnancies and one confinement by caesarean section in the past history). The pregnancy under review was non-developing, on 11th week, that ended surgically (curettage). Eight weeks after the curettage, haemorrhage occurred. The ultrasonography showed localized heterogeneous "aggregates" in the myometrium. The increased value of β-HCG in blood serum indicated at the presence of residual placental tissue. Diagnosis: placenta increta after abortion in the first trimester. Actions taken: transcatheter arterial chemoembolisation with dactinomycin for reaching immediate haemostasis and cellulicidal effect on placenta tissues. Twenty days after the chemoembolisation, the value of β-HCG in blood serum fell to the normal level, and the "aggregate" characterising impairment of the uterus according to the ultrasonography data disappeared without complications.

The clinical observation described by Chou et al. [39] in respect of a 35-year-old woman with continual vaginal haemorrhage and preceding caesarean section in anamnesis, demonstrated a diagnosed 7th week pregnancy. The ovum with dimensions of 2.5 × 1.5 cm was located within the area of a uterine scar from the previous caesarean section. The original treatment was one-time injection of Methotrexate. Nevertheless, β-HCG levels remained high, and the transvaginal ultrasonography showed signs of continuing pregnancy. Consequently, hysteroscopic resectoscopy

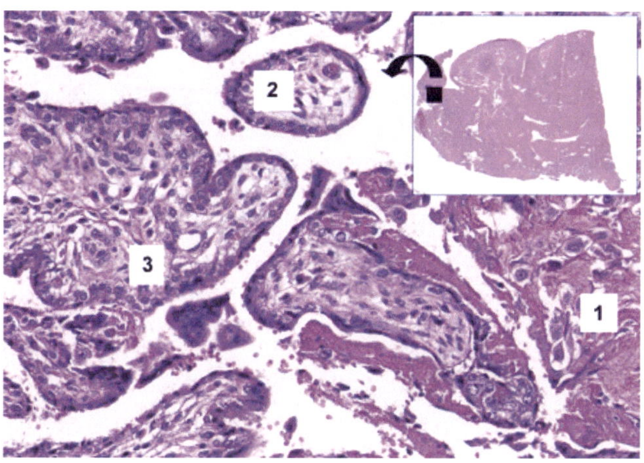

Figure 7.
Patient S., 40 years old. Diagnosis: pregnancy, 13 weeks. Caesarean section in the past medical history. Ingrowth of chorionic villi into the uterine scar. Laparotomy. It was found as wellas a fundal uterine defect of 4 ± 3 cm with placental tissue penetrating through the uterine serosa. Hysterectomy. Histology of the placenta showing the myometrium (1) with invasions of chorionic villi (2) and trophoblast cells (3) (x20; haematoxylin – eosin staining) [38].

was made during which the gestational tissue was completely removed. This did not entail any intra- or postoperative complications. The level of β-HCG in blood serum returned to normal 4 weeks after the operation. According to the authors, the hysteroscopic ectomy of ingrown chorion residues can be regarded as primary treatment, and as a secondary option-after an unsuccessful attempt of treatment with Methotrexate [39]. Histopathology of the placenta is shown in **Figure** 7, performed on a 40-year-old patient with a uterine rupture at 13 weeks of gestation, described by the authors A. Esmans et al. [38].

Lim et al. [24] give a clinical observation of placenta accreta and tardive haemorrhage in a patient aged 41 with five pregnancy episodes in the past medical history (1—confinement, 1—caesarean section for presentation of placenta and 3 curettage manipulations). Placenta accreta caused vaginal haemorrhage 3 years after the abortion, in the first trimester, 5 weeks' period. Originally the patient had regular menstruation, further the menses became irregular and heavy within the last year, which was the reason to seek medical attention. The level of serous β-HCG was 0.27 mIU/mL. The ultrasonography failed to visualize the endometrium line. Originally, endometrium cancer or uterine myoma with necrosis of the node was suspected. Actions taken: curettage; subsequently, in connection with the continuing haemorrhage-hysterectomy. The histopathological examination evidentiated the placenta tissue having no atypical trophoblast cells [24].

6. Recommendations for interruption of pregnancy in women with localisation of chorion/placenta in the uterine scar area after the caesarean section

The optimal treatment of patients in the first trimester of pregnancy with sonographic diagnosis of suspected chorion increta into the uterine scar remains uncertain. The suggested options include one principal type of treatment or its combination with other methods, like curettage, systemic or local administration of Methotrexate, hysteroscopy, laparotomy and uterine artery embolisation [22, 40].

A review by Timor-Tritsch and Monteagudo [22] analyses the structure of surgical interferences in 44 patients with the given diagnosis: 5 of them (10.6%) underwent uterine arteries embolisation; 38 (78.7%) were subjected to laparotomy; 35 of the latter (74.4%) to hysterectomy; 1 patient of this group was diagnosed with arteriovenous malformation after the dilation and curettage and was subjected to embolisation that subsequently ended in hysterectomy [22].

The sporadic, mainly individual, cases and their results are insufficient to draw a definite conclusion as to which of the performed interference methods is the most effective. It is almost impossible to identify what type of treatment entails maximum number of complications and should be avoided. Gynaecologists, as a rule, undertake curettage, laparoscopy and hysteroscopy, deeming them preferable as the "first-line" approach.

Nevertheless, the following recommendations were made on the basis of the meta-analysis [22]:

- If possible, dilation and curettage should be avoided because this might entail excessive bleeding, repeated curettage (for the haemostatic purpose) with no effect, blood transfusion, and in many cases—laparotomy and loss of uterus.

- Systemic administration of Methotrexate as the only method of treatment should be avoided. The argument: lengthy expectation of the effect or its absence results in further growth of the embryo and vascularisation of the gestational sac; therefore the subsequent, "second line" of therapy may be accompanied by considerable complications.

- Uterine artery embolisation as a primary treatment should be used cautiously or not be used at all. Lengthy expectation of haemostasis or the haemorrhage fadeout can delay more effective primary treatment which could help in a faster manner or might allow avoiding of hysterectomy.

- Surgical exsection of the impairment area through hysteroscopic method, as well as transvaginal or transabdominal local administration of Methotrexate with or without additional intramuscular dose of this medication, appears to be the optimal means in terms of minimisation of frequency of complications.

7. Conclusion

Interruption of pregnancy in case of a uterine scar can be effected at any pregnancy period using any method; at the same time, no additional risks for the mother are described if the ovum is localized beyond the scar zone.

Ultrasonic examination is an important method for viewing possible ovum presentation to the scar and possible chorion increta into the scar.

At suspicion on chorion ingrowth into the uterine scar, dilation and curettage, systemic administration of Methotrexate, uterine artery embolisation should be avoided, while it is recommended to give preference to combined methods—surgical exsection of the impairment zone through hysteroscopic access and local administration of Methotrexate.

In all cases, patients with the uterine scar (irrespective of localisation of the ovum) are subject to hospitalisation for interruption of pregnancy at any period.

Author details

Galina Dikke and Vladimir Ostromenskiy*
Academy of Medical Education Named After F.I. Inozemcev, Saint-Petersburg, Russia

*Address all correspondence to: ostromenskyvv@gmail.com

References

[1] Taha MS et al. Management of failed early pregnancies after previous multiple caesarean sections; an evolving clinical dilemma. EC Gynaecology. 2018;**7**(5):163-169

[2] Collins K, Alka K. Catastrophic consequences of a caesarean scar pregnancy missed on ultrasound. Australasian Journal of Ultrasound in Medicine. 2015;**18**(4):150-156

[3] Chen BA, Reeves MF, Creinin MD, Gilles JM, et al. Misoprostol for treatment of early pregnancy failure in women with prior uterine surgery. American Journal of Obstetrics and Gynecology. 2008;**198**(6):626e1-626e5

[4] Wang YL, Su TH, Huang WC, Weng SS. Laparoscopic management of placenta increta after late first-trimester dilation and evacuation manifesting as an unusual uterine mass. Journal of Minimally Invasive Gynecology. 2011;**18**(2):250-253

[5] Willmott FJ, Scherf C, Ford SM, Lim K. Rupture of uterus in the first trimester during medical termination of pregnancy for exomphalos using mifepristone/misoprostol. BJOG: An International Journal of Obstetrics and Gynaecology. 2008;**115**(12):1575-1577

[6] FIGO/Misoprostol. Recommended regimen. 2017. Available from: https://www.figo.org/

[7] Loïc S et al. Delivery for women with a previous caesarean: Guidelines for clinical practice from the French College of Gynecologists and Obstetricians (CNGOF). European Journal of Obstetrics, Gynecology, and Reproductive Biology. 2013;**170**(1):25-32

[8] NHS. Expectant Management of Miscarriage. 2012

[9] Allison JL et al. Management of first trimester pregnancy loss can be safely moved into the office. Reviews in Obstetrics and Gynecology. 2011;**4**(1):5-14

[10] Drezett J, Bessa MMM, Pedroso D, Silva ACF, et al. Misoprostol no aborto de segundo trimestre em gestações decorrentes de violência sexual: Análise de efetividade de um protocolo aplicado em serviço público de saúde brasileiro. Reprodução Climatério. 2014;**29**(3):105-111

[11] American College of Obstetricians and Gynecologists. Practice bulletin #135: Second-trimester abortion. Obstetrics and Gynecology. 2013;**121**:1394-1406

[12] Royal College of Obstetricians and Gynaecologists. The Care of Women Requesting Induced Abortion (Evidence-based Clinical Guideline No.7). London: RCOG Press; 2011. 130 p

[13] Maurer K, Jacobson J, Turok D. Same day cervical preparation with misoprostol prior to second trimester D&E: A case series. Contraception. 2013;**88**(1):116-121

[14] Hammond C, Chasen S. Dilation and evacuation. In: Paul M et al., editors. Management of Unintended and Abnormal Pregnancies: Comprehensive Abortion Care. Hoboken, USA: Wiley-Balckwell; 2009. pp. 157-177

[15] Borgatta L, Roncarib D, Sonalkara S, Mark A, et al. Mifepristone vs. osmotic dilator insertion for cervical preparation prior to surgical abortion at 14-16 weeks: A randomized trial. Contraception. 2012;86:567-557

[16] Lyus R, Lohr PA, Taylor J, Morroni C. Outcomes with same-day cervical preparation with Dilapan-S osmotic dilators and vaginal misoprostol before dilatation and evacuation at 18 to

21+6 weeks' gestation. Contraception. 2013;**87**(1):71-75

[17] Fox MC, Krajewski CM. Cervical preparation for second-trimester surgical abortion prior to 20 weeks' gestation: SFP clinical guidelines. Contraception. 2014;**89**:75-84

[18] Chambers DG, Willcourt RJ, Laver AR, Baird JK, Herbert WY. Comparison of Dilapan-S and laminaria for cervical priming before surgical pregnancy termination at 17-22 weeks' gestation. International Journal of Women's Health. 2011;**3**:347-352

[19] Rahimi-Sharbaf F, Jamal A, Mesdaghinia E, Abedzadeh-Kalahroudi M, et al. Ultrasound detection of placenta accreta in the first trimester of pregnancy. Iranian Journal of Reproductive Medicine. 2014;**12**(6):421-426

[20] Hudon L, Belfort MA, Broome DR. Diagnosis and management of placenta percreta: A review. Obstetrical & Gynecological Survey. 1998;**53**(8):509-517

[21] Wu S, Kocherginsky M, Hibbard JU. Abnormal placentation: Twenty-year analysis. American Journal of Obstetrics and Gynecology. 2005; **192**(5):1458-1461

[22] Timor-Tritsch IE, Monteagudo A. Unforeseen consequences of the increasing rate of caesarean deliveries: Early placenta accreta and caesarean scar pregnancy. American Journal of Obstetrics and Gynecology. 2012;**210**:371-374

[23] Abbas AM, Shymaa AM, Osama SA, Abdalmageed S. Placenta percreta presenting with marked hemoperitoneum in the first trimester of pregnancy: A case report. Middle East Fertility Society Journal. 2018;**23**(3):251-253. Available from: https://www.sciencedirect.com/

[24] Lim S, Ha SY, Lee KB, Lee JS. Retained placenta accreta after a first-trimester abortion manifesting as an uterine mass. Obstetrics & Gynecology Science. 2013;**56**(3):205-207

[25] Takeda A, Koyama K, Imoto S. Conservative management of placenta increta after first trimester abortion by transcatheter arterial chemoembolization: A case report and review of the literature. Archives of Gynecology and Obstetrics. 2010;**281**(3):381-386

[26] Jang DG, Lee GSR, Yoon JH, Lee SJ. Placenta percreta-induced uterine rupture diagnosed by laparoscopy in the first trimester: Case report. International Journal of Medical Sciences. 2011;**8**(5):424-427

[27] Patel MA. Scar ectopic pregnancy. Journal of Obstetrics and Gynaecology of India. 2015;**65**(6):372-375

[28] Dew L, Harris S, Yost N, Magee K, de Prisco G. Second trimester placenta percreta presenting as acute abdomen. Proceedings (Baylor University Medical Center). 2015;**28**(1):38-40

[29] Belfort MA. Placenta accreta. American Journal of Obstetrics and Gynecology. 2010;**203**(5):430-439

[30] Usta IM, Hobeika EM, Musa AA, Gabriel GE, Nassar AH. Placenta previa-accreta: Risk factors and complications. (Case-control level II-2). American Journal of Obstetrics and Gynecology. 2005;**193**:1045-1049

[31] Richardson A, Gallos I, Dobson S, Campbell BK, Coomarasamy A, Raine-Fenning N. Accuracy of first-trimester ultrasound in diagnosis of intrauterine pregnancy prior to visualization of the yolk sac: A systematic review and meta-analysis. Ultrasound in Obstetrics & Gynecology. 2015;**46**(2):142-149. DOI: 10.1002/uog

[32] Shawky M, AbouBieh E, Masood A. Gray scale and doppler ultrasound in placenta accreta: Optimization of ultrasound signs. Egyptian Journal of Radiology and Nuclear Medicine. 2016;**47**(3):1111-1115

[33] Twickler DM, Lucas MJ, Balis AB, Santos-Ramos R, Martin L, Malone S, et al. Color flow mapping for myometrial invasion in women with a prior caesarean delivery. The Journal of Maternal-Fetal Medicine. 2000;**9**(6):330-335

[34] Warshak CR, Eskander R, Hull AD, Scioscia AL, Mattrey RF, Benirschke K, et al. Accuracy of ultrasonography and magnetic resonance imaging in the diagnosis of placenta accreta. Obstetrics and Gynecology. 2006;**108** (3 Pt 1):573-581

[35] Varghese B, Singh N, George RAN, Gilvaz S. Magnetic resonance imaging of placenta accrete. Indian Journal of Radiology and Imaging. 2013;**23**(4):379-385

[36] Riteau AS, Tassin M, Chambon G, Le Vaillant C, de Laveaucoupet J, Quéré MP, et al. Accuracy of ultrasonography and magnetic resonance imaging in the diagnosis of placenta accreta. PLoS ONE. 2014;**9**(4):e94866. DOI: 10.1371/journal.pone.0094866

[37] Ju W, Kim SC. Placenta increta after first-trimester dilatation and curettage manifesting as an unusual uterine mass: Magnetic resonance findings. Acta Radiologica. 2007;**48**(8):938-940

[38] Esmans A, Gerris J, Corthout E, Verdonk P, Declercq S. Placenta percreta causing rupture of an unscarred uterus at the end of the first trimester of pregnancy: Case report. Human Reproduction. 2004;**19**(10):2401-2403

[39] Chou Y-M, Wu D, Wu K-Y, Lee C-L. Hysteroscopic removal of caesarean scar pregnancy after methotrexate treatment failure. Gynecology and Minimally Invasive Therapy. 2013;**2**(2):70-72. DOI: 10.1016/j.gmit.2013.02.008

[40] Boza A, Boza B, Api M. Caesarean scar pregnancy managed with conservative treatment. Iranian Journal of Medical Sciences. 2016;**41**:450-455